Pregnancy Fitness

Julia Di Paolo

Samantha Montpetit-Huynh

Kim Vopni

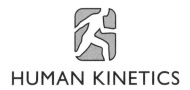

HUMAN KINETICS

Library of Congress Cataloging-in-Publication Data

Names: Paolo, Julia Di, 1973- author. | Montpetit-Huynh, Samantha, 1970-
author. | Vopni, Kim, author.
Title: Pregnancy fitness / Julia Di Paolo, Samantha Montpetit-Huynh, and Kim
Vopni.
Description: Champaign, IL : Human Kinetics, [2019] | Includes
bibliographical references and index. | Description based on print version record and CIP data provided
by publisher; resource not viewed.
Identifiers: LCCN 2017041810 (print) | LCCN 2017050915 (ebook) | ISBN
9781492552437 (ebook) | ISBN 9781492552420 (print)
Subjects: LCSH: Exercise for pregnant women. | Physical fitness for pregnant
women. | Pregnant women—Health and hygiene.
Classification: LCC RG558.7 (ebook) | LCC RG558.7 .P36 2019 (print) | DDC
618.2/44—dc23
LC record available at https://lccn.loc.gov/2017041810

ISBN: 978-1-4925-5242-0 (print)

This publication is written and published to provide accurate and authoritative information relevant to the subject matter presented. It is published and sold with the understanding that the author and publisher are not engaged in rendering legal, medical, or other professional services by reason of their authorship or publication of this work. If medical or other expert assistance is required, the services of a competent professional person should be sought.

The web addresses cited in this text were current as of November 2017, unless otherwise noted.

Acquisitions Editor: Diana Vincer; **Developmental Editor:** Laura Pulliam; **Managing Editor:** Ann C. Gindes; **Copyeditor:** Pamela S. Johnson; **Indexer:** Karla Walsh; **Permissions Manager:** Martha Gullo; **Graphic Designer:** Sean Roosevelt; **Cover Designer:** Keri Evans; **Cover Design Associate:** Susan Allen; **Photograph (cover):** © Human Kinetics; **Photographs (interior):** © Human Kinetics unless otherwise noted; **Illustrations:** © Human Kinetics; **Visual Production Assistant:** Joyce Brumfield; **Photo Production Manager:** Jason Allen; **Senior Art Manager:** Kelly Hendren; **Printer:** Edwards Brothers Malloy

We thank Yoga Star Studio in Toronto, Canada, for assistance in providing the location for the photo shoot for this book.

Human Kinetics books are available at special discounts for bulk purchase. Special editions or book excerpts can also be created to specification. For details, contact the Special Sales Manager at Human Kinetics.

Printed in the United States of America   10 9 8 7 6 5 4 3 2 1

The paper in this book is certified under a sustainable forestry program.

Human Kinetics
P.O. Box 5076
Champaign, IL 61825-5076
Website: www.HumanKinetics.com

In the United States, e-mail info@hkusa.com or call 800-747-4457.
In Canada, e-mail info@hkcanada.com.
In the United Kingdom/Europe, e-mail hk@hkeurope.com.

For information about Human Kinetics' coverage in other areas of the world,
please visit our website: **www.HumanKinetics.com**

E7085

Pregnancy Fitness

We are continuously inspired and driven forward by all our clients and patients, especially the ones who ask, "Why didn't anyone tell me about this *before* I got pregnant?" We dedicate this book to all the women who are currently pregnant and to those who may become pregnant in the future. Our sincere hope is that you use the information in this book to prepare, recover, and restore. Take action, prepare your body for birth, honor your postpartum recovery, and then tell others what you have learned. Together we can help everyone have a better birth and recovery and enjoy core confidence for motherhood!

CONTENTS

Part III Sample Programs for Each Phase of Pregnancy

EXERCISE FINDER

(continued)

(continued)

PREFACE

When a woman becomes a mother, it is a transformative time in her life. It is a time when with significant changes occur in the mind, body, and spirit. Cultures around the world honor this time with various traditions that often focus on rest, nourishment, and support for the new mother so she can transition to her new role with ease. In Japan it is customary for the new mother to rest for three weeks and stay in bed in her parents' home. In Nigeria the tradition of *Omugwo*, which means postpartum care, calls for the grandmother to give the new baby his or her first bath. This shows the mother that she is supported and has a village to help with child rearing. In Latin America, *la cuarentena* (the quarantine) is a six-week period in which new mothers abstain from sex, strenuous activity, and certain foods. They dedicate themselves simply to rest, healing, and breastfeeding. They are supported by their family members, who cook, clean, and care for the other children and the new baby.

In North America we lack traditions related to healing practices in pregnancy and the postpartum period. Unfortunately, our society and media encourage a super-mom mentality that applauds a quick return to fitness and promotes the goal of looking "like you never had a baby."

Our goal with this book is to play a role in creating a paradigm shift that introduces cultural traditions to the Western world; such traditions would be instrumental in improving birth outcomes, promoting the need for a purposeful recovery, and revering the women who choose a gradual return to exercise.

We are believers in movement during pregnancy, childbirth, and motherhood, and we stress the importance of moving with awareness. Our passion is educating pregnant women and the professionals who work with them about the many changes that pregnancy and childbirth bring. Knowledge is power; when women are in a position of power, they can make informed choices about their bodies during pregnancy, childbirth, and motherhood.

First, we will explore the effects of pregnancy on the body and give you an understanding of what to expect, how to manage the changes, and how to move in ways that respect the changes while still maintaining your fitness.

Next, we will introduce the concept of being fit for childbirth. Most people understand the concept of preparing for a race or a climb; any physical event needs physical preparation. Well, birth is a very physical event—one that we believe a mother should train for. We are excited to show you how!

The pelvic floor and abdomen are our areas of specialty, and these are two topics that we see left out of many prenatal education programs. The pelvic floor and the abs are on the minds of all expectant women, and we want you to know how to support your core and pelvic floor during pregnancy, childbirth, and your recovery so you have the body confidence you deserve in motherhood.

Once we have educated you on the changes that happen, we want you to know how to move! *Pregnancy Fitness* is all about you moving in ways that prepare your body for birth and optimize your recovery. We guide you through exercises that can be used as part of your workouts to keep your core and pelvic floor safe and ready for the task at hand. We have exercises for the upper body, exercises for the lower body, and functional exercises that get you ready for motherhood, as well as stretching and release work that will help you let go of tension and holding patterns that often contribute to aches and pains or challenges in labor.

Finally, we give you actual workouts for each trimester. These workouts are designated according to fitness level—beginner, intermediate, and advanced—so no matter what your current level is or when in your pregnancy you find this book, you will have the plan that is right for you. We designed the workouts with the demands of each trimester in mind so that you will be strong, confident, and ready for the big day!

We put a lot of love and energy into this book, and we are grateful that you found this text and are putting our work into practice. We wish you an informed and empowered pregnancy, birth, and recovery.

ACKNOWLEDGMENTS

We would like to acknowledge the following individuals (in no particular order) for inspiring and educating us.

Diane Lee

Julie Wiebe

Julie Tupler

All our patients and clients

Nadine Woods

Each other

Our husbands and children

Marie Josee Lord and Claudia Brown

Nelly Faghani

Carolyn Van Dyken

Andrea Page

Dr. Bruce Crawford

Tom Myers

Jenny Burrell

Katy Bowman

Kristina Bosnar

Sue Dumais

Dr. Marjorie Dixon

Dr. Jon Barrett

Paul Hodges

Stu McGill

Dr. Herb Wong

canfitpro

Jill Miller

Our master trainers

All the researchers who have taken time to study and publish their work

Understanding Your Body Through Pregnancy

Effects of Pregnancy

Pregnancy is an exciting time full of anticipation and preparation. It is also a time of significant change in the body. There are hormonal changes; posture and alignment changes; muscle, ligament, and tissue changes as well as respiratory and energy-level changes. There is a lot for the body to do in order to grow a new life, and all the changes to the body can also affect the mind and spirit of an expectant mother. Your mind is probably working overtime these days, with so much to learn and do that it can often be overwhelming. Energy-level fluctuations, body-image concerns, and uncertainties of motherhood are all realities to be faced. Compounding that fact is the upcoming due date, which can contribute to feelings of anxiety and fear. It is well known that exercise helps manage stress and can improve moods. Exercise is essential for everyone but especially for pregnant women, because it better enables the body to grow a healthy baby, manage the changes that are occurring, and quiet the mind.

There is no question that pregnancy brings some very visible changes to the body. Larger breasts and an ever-growing belly are the two most obvious, but there is also a lot going on inside that you can't see. Subtle changes to posture and alignment, hormone-level changes, increased stretch of certain muscles and tissues, and a shifting center of gravity are just a few of the less-visible changes. Movement and exercise are essential to help ensure these changes do not result in excessive weight gain, gestational diabetes, or pain and discomfort. A review of available data consistently shows women who exercise in their pregnancies reduce their risk of gestational diabetes by almost 50% and their risk of developing preeclampsia by almost 40%. Any moderate exercise during pregnancy reduced the risk of gestational diabetes by more than 30 percent, and if the exercise was done throughout the entire pregnancy that percentage dropped another 6 percent (Dempsey, Butler, and Williams 2005).

Furthermore, the endorphins released during exercise provide positive psychological effects, which is especially helpful with all the physical changes that are happening. Exercise should be considered an essential part of preparing for the birth as well. While the process of labor and birth is often portrayed as passive (a woman lying on a bed), it is really quite a dynamic, active event. Just like any other physical event, the more someone has trained for it, the better she will perform.

Let's look more closely at the effects of pregnancy on the body and how you can use exercise to support your body in pregnancy and best prepare for labor and birth.

HORMONAL CHANGES

It is no secret that hormones play significant roles in conception, pregnancy, labor, and the postpartum body. In this section, we will look at the main hormones that affect the pregnant body most profoundly. We have not listed all the hormones, because we are focusing on those that contribute most to the changes.

Human Chorionic Gonadotropin (HCG)

This hormone is secreted in your urine and is used by home pregnancy tests to determine if you are pregnant. The role of HCG is to tell your body that there is a life form in your womb and that your body needs to get ready to nurture it. HCG also tells the ovaries to stop maturing an egg every month. The level of HCG rises consistently until it reaches a peak around the end of the first trimester, which typically coincides with an end to the nausea as well. While the cause of morning sickness has never been determined with 100 percent agreement, many health professionals believe it is HCG. This hormone is also responsible for increasing the blood supply to the pelvis, which can make the signal to empty the bladder increase in frequency.

Exercise can be a challenge in the early weeks and months of pregnancy because of the nausea. Gentle walks, release work (such as stretching and yoga), and light weight training, as tolerated, are all great options to choose until you are feeling better. Some women find fresh air and movement can help ease the symptoms while others simply can't make it far from the bathroom.

Nausea is the most common reason women may need to stick close to a toilet, but if it is the increase in bladder signals that keeps you close to the bathroom, recognize that it is not always because your bladder is full. A bladder should signal to empty every two-and-a-half to four hours. In pregnancy, whether because of hormones or because of reduced space and more pressure on the bladder, the signal to empty may come more often. This can in turn train the bladder to continue to signal before it is completely full even after you are no longer pregnant. Once your baby is born, ensure you work to retrain your bladder so it knows it is not okay to want to empty every 45 to 60 minutes. We will talk more about this in chapter 3.

Progesterone

Progesterone keeps the uterus muscle relaxed by inhibiting it from contracting. Progesterone also plays a role in the immune system by helping the body tolerate foreign DNA (the fetus). Early on, progesterone is produced by the corpus luteum in the ovary. By the second trimester, it switches to being produced by the placenta. Progesterone contributes to relaxation of the blood vessels throughout the body, which can contribute to lower-than-normal blood pressure. Because it also relaxes all smooth muscles such as the intestines, the passage of food through the intestines can slow down and contribute to constipation.

Constipation is an unpleasant side effect of progesterone. It is uncomfortable and can lead to straining, which can be damaging to the pelvic floor (the group of muscles at the base of the pelvis). The pelvic floor will undergo a lot of strain during childbirth, so you don't want to experience additional strain on a daily basis due to constipation. Be sure you stay well hydrated and eat high-fiber foods (both soluble and insoluble fiber) to help make your bowel movements easy to pass. Exercise and movement can also help with constipation, so aim to get out for a daily walk. Walking is also beneficial for the pelvic floor and of course for mental well-being. Emotional stress and the decrease in blood pressure may cause tiredness, so pay attention to how you are feeling.

During pregnancy, the general feeling of exhaustion, as well as a feeling of breathlessness brought on by what used to be a very easy task, can be attributed to progesterone. Progesterone makes your body extra sensitive to carbon dioxide in your blood and actually causes you to breathe more deeply so that the oxygen demands for you and baby are met.

The early influence of progesterone can often make the first trimester a big challenge physically, mentally, and emotionally. For active women, feeling sick, tired, and constipated all the time is a struggle, and many women just want it to be over so they can feel like themselves again.

Take Action

Managing the hormonal roller coaster and the mood swings in pregnancy can be challenging. Prenatal massage can work wonders at reducing stress hormones (cortisol and norepinephrine) and increasing serotonin and dopamine levels (the "feel good" hormones). We all have varying levels of these even when we are not pregnant, but pregnancy worries can contribute to higher levels of the stress hormones. When added to the other hormonal fluctuations, many women feel like they are just not quite themselves. Prenatal massage not only feels good physically but also can help you feel good emotionally as well. It helps stabilize hormone levels and may even help reduce the likelihood of depression (Field, Figueiredo, Hernandez-Reif, Diego, Dees, and Ascencio 2008).

Estrogen

Estrogen production occurs only in the ovaries in early pregnancy and then switches to the placenta by the second trimester. Estrogen levels rise slowly and consistently throughout pregnancy until estrogen starts to be produced more quickly as the end of the pregnancy approaches. The role of estrogen is to help stimulate hormone production in the fetus's adrenal gland, stimulate growth of the fetus's adrenal gland, and prepare and enhance your uterus so it can respond to oxytocin when the time comes to birth your baby. Elevated estrogen levels may not only prompt nausea but also may increase your appetite.

During the second trimester, estrogen plays a major role in the milk duct development that enlarges the breasts. As the breasts become larger in pregnancy, posture and alignment change. The pelvis may start to tip anteriorly, the shoulders start to round, and you may start to lean back to counteract the shifting center of gravity. Ensure you have a well-fitting maternity bra and make a point to check your posture several times throughout the day. Try to do lots of stretching and release work to open the chest, lengthen the hamstrings, and stretch the hips.

Relaxin

Relaxin is a hormone produced by the ovaries and the placenta that is responsible for relaxing the ligaments in the pelvis as well as softening and lengthening the cervix. Relaxin is often blamed for the aches and pains commonly associated with pregnancy. You may feel less stable in all joints, most markedly in the pelvis. Relaxin is at its highest in the first trimester and at delivery. It is not known exactly how long relaxin levels stay elevated in the body after the baby is born, but it is typically present from four to nine months postpartum.

BODY FACT

In pregnancy, the linea alba will often turn brown. Then, it is called the linea nigra ("black line"). This dark vertical line appears on the abdomen in approximately three quarters of all pregnancies. The brownish line runs vertically along the midline of the abdomen from the pubis to the umbilicus, but can also run from the pubis to the top of the abdomen. During pregnancy, increased melanocyte-stimulating hormone made by the placenta causes the line to darken. The hormone also contributes to melasma (darker areas of skin, also called "the mask of pregnancy") and darkened nipples.

The linea alba (LA), which means "white line," is another area of the body that is sensitive to the increase in relaxin. The LA is the connective tissue that holds the two straps of the rectus abdominis (the "6-pack" muscles) in place. As the uterus grows, the LA must expand to accommodate the growing baby, which causes the two straps of the rectus abdominis to move away from the midline of the body. This is termed diastasis rectus abdominis. You may also see it written as diastasis recti or simply DRA. Recent research has determined that 100 percent of women will get this abdominal separation by the 35th week of pregnancy. More on this can be found in chapter 4.

Movement, especially movement with awareness, is essential during pregnancy. With the knowledge that your pelvis is less stable and your abs are shifting out of their ideal alignment, you can make more appropriate exercise choices that safeguard and build up your body rather than put it at increased risk for injury.

BODY CHANGES

The influence of hormones contributes to many of the changes your body is going through; however, other systems in the body are undergoing change as well. Just like your baby grows and develops each day, so do you! Pregnancy is a constant state of change and adaptation that culminates in the birth of your baby. Let's look at some of the other changes that are happening in your body and some ways to help adjust.

Cardiovascular System Changes

Your pregnant body must work harder to circulate oxygen and blood around your body. Your heart rate will fluctuate with the changes you encounter in each trimester. Early on, your resting heart rate will increase by about 10 to 20 beats per minute. This means that your exercising heart rate will also be higher. This increase is caused by hormonal changes, including those that cause vasodilation (widening of the blood vessels). As a result of this widening, the blood pressure drops so your pregnant body must work harder to circulate oxygen and blood throughout a larger surface area. Over time, your body will adapt and your exercising heart rate may return to closer to what it was before you were pregnant. During pregnancy, monitoring your exertion level by how fast your heart is beating is not as reliable. The talk test and the rate of perceived exertion (RPE) are better for determining a suitable intensity level for exercise. The RPE is a scale to help you determine the intensity of your exercise (see table 1.1).

Mentally, feeling winded can be a challenge for many women, especially those who considered themselves fit before pregnancy. Many women say they suddenly feel out of shape, which can be discouraging to those who felt they were at their peak of physical fitness before getting pregnant.

Table 1.1 Rating of Perceived Exertion (RPE) Scale

RPE number	Breathing rate / ability to talk	Exertion
1	Resting	Very slight
2	Talking is easy	Slight
3	Talking is easy	Moderate
4	You can talk but with more effort	Somewhat hard
5	You can talk but with more effort	Hard
6	Breathing is challenged/don't want to talk	Hard
7	Breathing is challenged/don't want to talk	Very hard
8	Panting hard/conversation is difficult	Very, very hard
9	Panting hard/conversation is difficult	Very, very hard
10	Cannot sustain this intensity for too long	Maximal

Reprinted, by permission, from K. Austin and B. Seebohar, 2011, *Performance nutrition: Applying the science of nutrient timing* (Champaign IL: Human Kinetics), 30.

Around the midpoint of pregnancy, when progesterone relaxes the walls of the blood vessels and contributes to lowering the blood pressure, some women may feel faint if they stand too long or if they get up too quickly. Pregnancy and birth are very physical events, and looking at them as though they are another event to train for can help bring a more positive outlook. We'll discuss this training and heart rate monitoring in chapter 2.

Respiratory System Changes

Early on in pregnancy, hormonal changes typically contribute to feelings of breathlessness. Even though you are actually getting more oxygen into your system, it sure doesn't feel like it! As the pregnancy progresses and the uterus moves up out of the pelvis, the space into which the diaphragm descends when you inhale decreases, which can make it difficult to take a deep breath. The pressure of the uterus on the diaphragm increases the work required for breathing, because it is harder for the diaphragm to contract and descend on the inhalation. Therefore, more effort and energy are required to bring in the same amount of air. This can mean less oxygen is available for aerobic exercise.

Making sure you stand and move frequently throughout the day will help offset these effects, as will stretching and muscle release work for the side body and obliques. When tension is held in the rib cage or the obliques, it can restrict the expansion of the ribs and descent of the diaphragm needed during inhalation. Even later in pregnancy, when the uterus is starting to limit the contraction of the diaphragm, having freedom in the obliques can help you bring in more air.

Skeletal Alignment Changes

It is no surprise that the growth of the abdomen in pregnancy causes shifts in the center of gravity. When not pregnant, your weight should be more over your heels, meaning your pelvis should be over your ankles and your ribs should be over your pelvis. As the belly grows, there is a greater mass out front that can start to alter your center of gravity, but ideally, you should still be able to keep your pelvis over your ankles. Unfortunately, our modern-day lifestyle, with increased sitting and lack of walking and squatting, means our backsides typically don't have the mass to counterbalance the growing belly. The result is compensations in the form of tight hamstrings, the pelvis migrating forward in front of the ankles, flat gluteal muscles that don't work like they should, and pelvic floor muscles that are short and tight. The exercise sections will cover key release work and movements that will help ensure your backside can counterbalance the front to keep you in optimal alignment. The proper movement and release work can enable your body to better carry the weight of your baby with less strain on the ligaments, making the experience more comfortable while also encouraging optimal fetal positioning (see figure 1.1).

In ideal alignment, there would be a plumb line that would run in a straight line from the ears through the shoulders, hips, knees and ankles. There are apps that allow you to use your photo and apply a plumb line to see how well or not aligned you are. For a quick glimpse, you can use a strap or a card with a weight on the end, like the buckle on the end of a yoga strap, and hold it close to your pelvis with the weighted end hanging at your ankles. Simply hold the strap where your greater trochanter bulges on the outside of your thigh at your hip and allow the weight of the buckle end to point out where you are holding your weight. Ideally, the buckle will be beside the ankle, but for those whose weight is more forward, the buckle will hang closer to the center or front part of the foot. This allows you to see where your pelvis is in relation to your ankles and can provide some good insight into how you hold your body in space.

The growth of the breasts is another pull on the frame that can contribute to the body finding different strategies for balance and control. As the breasts grow, the heaviness can encourage rounding of the shoulders. Rather than accepting this change as being caused by the enlarged breasts, we should look at addressing tightness in the chest and weakness in the upper back—issues that can be easily tackled throughout pregnancy—to mitigate the alterations to alignment.

The feet often give us clues to changes up above. Some women claim that their feet grow in pregnancy. What may really be happening is that weakness in the lateral hip rotators cause the thighs to rotate internally, which in turn can cause the arches to lower. It may also be that hormonal

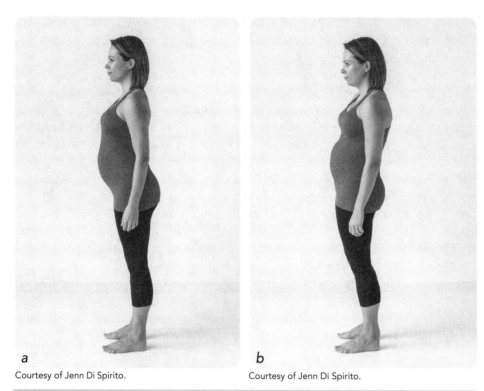

a

Courtesy of Jenn Di Spirito.

b

Courtesy of Jenn Di Spirito.

Figure 1.1   Compare (a) good alignment versus (b) poor alignment in pregnancy. Notice in the image on the right (b) how the weight has shifted forward over the forefoot.

BODY FACT

The stability of our joints is maintained by ligaments that allow articular motion. Ligaments are tough yet flexible fibrous bands of connective tissue. In pregnancy, relaxin increases the water content of collagen fibers in the ligaments, which increases their elasticity. These more supple and pliable ligaments allow for more movement of the bony structures, which is needed during the birth process, but it also reduces stability in the joints and can contribute to changes in alignment, leading to pain and vulnerability in pregnancy.

changes contribute to the ligamentous arch in the foot softening, especially when the center of gravity pulls the weight of the body more to the forefoot (in front of the ankle). This can create the illusion of the foot being longer. Choosing exercise and movements that work on the lateral rotators of the hip will help, as will spending more time "barefoot and pregnant" so that the muscles in the foot work as they should rather than being restricted by the shoes you wear.

Abdominal Changes

As we have mentioned, the abdominal wall is one part of the body that undergoes a lot of change and contributes to the shifting center of gravity. This can in turn start to affect the alignment of the pelvis and cause the body to utilize compensatory strategies to find and maintain stability.

With the pull of the growing abdomen, the tendency is for the top of the pelvis to start to tip anteriorly (forward), resulting in a more significant curve in the lumbar spine (the low back). As pregnancy progresses, the natural reaction to the heaviness in front and the pelvis tipping forward is to lean back and press the entire pelvis forward. Over time, this can result in a loss of the lumbar curve (the gentle curve in the low back) and a non-optimal curve higher in the spine. It can also contribute to a tight posterior pelvic floor, and glutes that no longer work as they should. This is not at all what we presented as optimal alignment with the ribs over the pelvis and the pelvis over the ankles. See figure 1.2 for an example of an abnormal curve.

Many women are not aware of the subtle alignment shifts and think it is normal to have aches and pains in pregnancy. With the right body awareness, education, and daily movement, pregnancy can be comfortable and alignment can be maintained close to normal even with the shifts in the center of gravity. The key is to move with awareness, release tension around the pelvis, and ensure that you work on the glutes throughout pregnancy. This will allow the baby to grow "in" the body rather than "out in front," so there will be less change in the center of gravity and less strain on the abdominal wall.

In pregnancy, the abdomen goes from being relatively flat to being convex with obvious stretching of the muscles and connective tissue, namely the linea alba. The stretching of the linea alba contributes to the condition diastasis recti (introduced briefly earlier in this chapter but covered in more detail in chapter 4). While diastasis recti is a normal response to pregnancy, it is worth taking steps to minimize it so that the abdominal wall has a better opportunity to return to optimal function postpartum. Studies have shown that over 50 percent of women with diastasis recti have some form of pelvic floor dysfunction such as incontinence or prolapse (Spitznagle, Leong, and Van Dillen 2007). The rectus muscles attach to the pubic symphysis (the pubic joint or pubic bone as most people call it), so it only makes sense that if the muscles have stretched or moved out of their normal anatomical position, the pelvis may be affected.

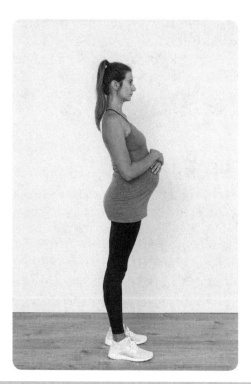

Figure 1.2   Abnormal lumbar curve in pregnancy.

When the pelvic floor and the muscles around the pelvis, such as the psoas, have normal tone, there is space for the baby to be "in" the pelvis. When the pelvic floor and the psoas muscles have too much tone or are tight and holding tension, it can mean less space in the pelvis. In turn, the abdomen will expand farther out in front, creating more strain on the linea alba. This increases the chances of the recti muscles moving farther away from the midline and presents a greater challenge for the connective tissue to regain its normal tension, which stabilizes the core.

When talking about changes in the abdomen, we need to address the psychological and emotional sides too. While the first signs of the baby bump can be exciting, as the pregnancy progresses and the belly gets bigger and bigger, thoughts turn to "how am I going to get my abs back?" It can be unsettling, especially if you have been quite fit, to gain weight and watch your body change. The exercises in this book, along with the awareness about body alignment that you will put into practice, are all designed to optimize your body and ensure your abs *will* return to optimal form and function so you will have confidence in your postpartum body and your journey into motherhood.

Take Action

The more modernized our world becomes, the more time we spend sitting. Many people sit for the majority of the day, usually in terrible posture. Most people sit on their sacrum (the triangle-shape bone in your pelvis that joins with the tailbone) rather than on their sitz bones (the two bony prominences you can feel in your butt if you pull the flesh in your butt cheeks apart). This posture chronically contracts and shortens the pelvic floor, therefore reducing space in the pelvis—the opposite of what you want when it comes time to birth your baby. This position also moves the pelvic floor out of its optimal alignment with the diaphragm. Sitting also shortens the hamstrings and, if you wear heeled shoes, your calves as well. If you must sit, do so with a neutral pelvis and sit for no more than one hour at a time. Take regular breaks to stretch and move to lengthen your calves and hamstrings and allow your pelvic floor to "breathe." If you really can't get up and move, then at the very least change your sitting posture frequently. We aren't saying you can never slouch; we are just suggesting that it is not ideal to spend the majority of your day in that position.

Alignment Check

When standing, ensure your feet are pelvis-width apart. Note we said pelvis width, not hip width. To see the difference, stand and put your fingers on your "hip bones" on the front of your pelvis. These bony prominences, called anterior superior iliac spines, or ASIS for short, should line up with the middle of the top of your feet. That is pelvis width. Now back your pelvis up so that your perineum (the area between your vagina and anus) is over the space between your ankle bones. Remember the plumb line self-assessment? You can use your plumb line and assess each time you stand. The more you stand correctly, the less you will need to check your plumb line. Next, now that your pelvis is backed up, you need to release tension in the glutes and posterior pelvic floor. Imagine "blossoming" your butt cheeks. Think of a flower opening and blooming: now apply that image to your butt cheeks. Once your pelvis is backed up and your buttocks are blossomed, check in with your ribs—are they over the pelvis? Many people have a tendency to hide their poor posture by pushing the ribs forward and getting military in their upper back. Instead, you should soften and drop your ribs so that they are stacked over your pelvis and your pelvis is over your ankles. Try to check in with your alignment several times a day, and soon you will be spending more and more time well aligned.

(continued)

Take Action   *(continued)*

Meditation and Visualization

Get to know your pelvis and pelvic floor. Understand that the baby comes out of the vagina and that the vagina will expand and that the bony attachment points of the pelvic floor can be visualized as a door. The pelvic door needs to be able to open freely to facilitate birth. Learn to release tension and create space between the pubic symphysis (the pubic bone), the tailbone, and the two sitz bones (those bony protrusions you can feel in each butt cheek). Take time each day to meditate and visualize softening around your pelvis so your pelvic door will open with ease on the big day.

Your amazing body is going through some pretty significant changes and will continue to do so as your pregnancy progresses. Developing an awareness of the changes, why they are happening, and how you can best support your body through those changes will go a long way toward optimizing your birth *and* your recovery. From hormonal to biomechanical changes and more, you will experience an incredible process as you grow and ready yourself to birth your baby. In the next chapter, we will look at exercise and movement in pregnancy while keeping all these changes in mind.

2

Get Fit for Birth

To truly be fit for birth, you need to move in ways that prepare you for the big day. That doesn't mean just exercising, but increasing your movement in general. We live in a world where we can and often choose to outsource much of our movement. While this might seem like a great idea, our bodies—especially when pregnant—really like to move! Instead, we use automatic doors, escalators, and moving sidewalks, and we drive almost daily, usually to an office where we sit most of the day. Because of this, we perform very little natural movement and ultimately rely on our one-hour exercise classes to convince ourselves that we are fit. But what are we fit for? Birth is an active and dynamic process. The popular media has done a good job of portraying birth as something you do lying on your back, but birthing a baby is not something to be "taken lying down." The more upright and mobile you are, the easier your baby will move into and out of your pelvis. Movements and fitness activities that take into account the changes happening in pregnancy, that mimic labor, and that blend strength and release work are the best choices to help you stay fit in pregnancy and get fit for birth.

Labor, birth, and motherhood offer many physical and emotional challenges, so when you move and exercise in ways that prepare you for those challenges, well, they become a bit less challenging. Be deliberate in your daily activities and find ways to sit less and move more; choose exercise that helps prepare your body for the big day and for your new role as a mother. Motherhood requires you to move in ways that you may not be accustomed to: carrying uneven, heavy loads (car seats and laundry baskets); bending and lifting (placing baby in car seats and cribs); twisting and rotating (calming a fussy baby in the car); and sometimes carrying laundry in one arm while carrying and calming a fussy baby with the other! Let's delve deeper and look at best practices for preparing the body for birth and motherhood.

THE PRINCIPLE OF SPECIFICITY

The principle of specificity is nothing new in the fitness realm but it is remarkable that, until recently, the principle has not been applied to pregnancy and birth. It has been understood that staying active during pregnancy is beneficial and being fit can improve the birth process and speed postpartum recovery. Unfortunately, research leading to recommendations for specific training for the event of childbirth has been overlooked.

As an active woman who is now pregnant, you appreciate the need to stay fit and you most likely have a strong desire to return to your pre-pregnancy fitness level once your baby is born. You may have begun your search for safe exercises or information about intensity levels, but do you really know how to train for the demands of birth?

Fitness and movement play an undeniably important role in childbirth. It stands to reason that training the pregnant body using movements that mimic labor and birth could contribute to better births and recoveries for many women. Childbirth is a physically demanding event that requires a balance between effort and surrender. It requires endurance, strength, flexibility, and a mind–body connection that ensures that the body responds appropriately, meaning it can soften, let go of tension, and allow labor and birth to unfold. Therefore, training the entire body is essential, and the elements of training, recovery, and retraining are key just as they are for any other physical event you may have trained for in the past.

In recent years, the trend in sports and fitness is to make workouts and training increasingly more intense. This type of challenging workout is attractive to many pregnant women, especially to new moms who feel out of shape after being pregnant and just want to feel like themselves again.

While birth is a very physically demanding event, we need to concentrate on specificity. What does the body need to do in labor and birth and what movements and exercises will train the body for the big day? The key is not to reach for 1-rep max goals or to set speed or distance goals but rather to move in ways that challenge the body now and work to prepare the body for labor and birth. Box jumps are not required in birth; nor are medicine ball slams or mountain climbers. While those exercises can certainly build up strength and endurance, are they actually preparing the body for birth? It's understandable if you are an avid CrossFitter and can't imagine not participating in your daily workout, but perhaps with the information in this book you may choose to modify your current workout regimen and set a goal to be back at it after your baby is born and when your core has been retrained and restored.

Fitness training should be specific to the demands of birth and specific to the needs of each trimester, including the fourth trimester—the recovery period. Your training will vary through the trimesters to ensure your body is ready for what lies ahead. Early on, the focus is on your core. When you reach the second trimester, strength and endurance using both cardiovascular training and muscular training are key components. Then, in the third trimester, both strength and endurance training continue, but the intensity is dialed back and more attention is paid to release work, stretching, and visualization as well as learning functional movements for motherhood. The exercises in this book will help you prepare your body for motherhood with movements like deadlifts, squats, and one-arm carries—moves you will be doing many times every day. Finally, the priority of the fourth trimester is healing, recovering, retraining, and restoring using many of the exercises you perfected in pregnancy. Let's face it, as a new mom you won't want to have to learn a new exercise program on top of learning to how breastfeed, care for a new baby, and do it all on very little sleep.

As you might already know, all workouts, training regimens, and exercise programs include a recovery component. Rest is an essential element of training, yet new moms often do too much too soon and make poor decisions regarding their return to exercise. They fail to take the time to recover from birth and to gradually retrain their body. They jump right back into what they were doing before they were pregnant and give no thought at all to the changes the body underwent in pregnancy or the fact that birth leaves the body in a somewhat injured state that needs time to heal (much longer than six weeks). A researcher at Salford University in England interviewed women at different stages of postpartum and found that it can take a full year to recover from childbirth (Wray 2011). By six weeks postpartum, initial tissue healing will be well under way, and the uterus will usually have returned to its non-pregnant state. But it will take your whole body much longer to achieve full recovery.

TYPES OF TRAINING

Fitness has several elements, and each affects different systems of your body. There is muscular strength and endurance, cardiovascular endurance, flexibility, muscle release and relaxation and functional movement to improve activities of daily living. No element alone is sufficient for fitness; all play important roles in your overall health and well-being. Depending on your goal, the activities you choose as part of your training program will be reflective of what you are training for. Someone training for a marathon, for example, will need to build up her cardiovascular endurance. That doesn't mean she'll work on only that element. The other elements play key roles as well, and each workout will have aspects of all of them, with the major focus being on cardiovascular endurance. The goal of a successful pregnancy and birth is not a set amount of time or distance as it is with a marathon. As an event, labor and birth is not a consistent environment: each woman's experience is different, as is each pregnancy and birth. Your training in pregnancy should cover all elements of fitness to help you build a body that is strong yet supple and able to go the distance.

Muscular Strength and Endurance

Early on in pregnancy is a great time to really focus on building and maintaining a strong core. The core is made up of the pelvic floor, the diaphragm (the muscle that controls breathing), the multifidus (deep spinal muscles), and the transversus abdominis muscles (the deepest abdominal muscles). These four key components make up what is called the "Core 4," and they need to work synergistically to support the body in movement. As the pregnancy progresses, many changes affect the Core 4 as it responds to an ever-increasing load. The pelvic floor has additional weight to adjust to, the abdominals undergo an ever-increasing stretch, the center of gravity shifts, and the muscles in the back face additional strain. Building a strong and functional Core 4 early on in pregnancy can help minimize the shifts in gravity, the strain on the back, and the stretch of the abdominals and ensure the pelvic floor is well-positioned to handle the increasing weight of the baby. The next chapter will present more detail about the Core 4.

Body alignment and posture are key to enabling the core to respond to the demands of pregnancy. Breath work such as the core breath (you will learn more about how the core breath relates to the abdominals in chapter 4 and a step-by-step exercise in chapter 6) is a daily essential that will train the core functionally in preparation for birth. The core breath is also the first exercise you will do after your baby is born to optimize your recovery and kick-start your core retraining. Starting core breathing in pregnancy takes advantage of creating muscle memory so that when you use it to restore and retrain postpartum, your body already knows what to do and you will recover more efficiently and quickly. Applying the core breath to dynamic movement is a fantastic birth prep workout too! This will be covered in depth in the exercise section in chapter 6.

While strengthening the core is essential, so too is building endurance of both body and mind. Birth is often compared to a marathon, but it makes more sense to compare it to three or four back to back marathons or an Ironman! Marathons last between two to eight hours, but most labors are much longer than that—sometimes an entire day or even two. A strong

BODY FACT

The amount of air moving into and out of your lungs in pregnancy increases by about 50 percent because each breath contains a greater volume of air and the rate of breathing increases. In the second and third trimesters, when the uterus is larger (and growing larger each day), the downward movement of the diaphragm with each inhale may be limited. This is why some women report feeling like it is more difficult to take deep breaths.

mind and body that have the mental and physical stamina to endure the challenge is vital. Increased sets and repetitions in your workouts is one way to prepare. Daily practice of birth positions and using visualization are two others. Just as an athlete would visualize the event, you should envision your labor and birth and help pattern your brain to be ready for the big day. In chapter 6, we will discuss visualization. Chapters 7, and 8, will go into detail about exercises, sets, and reps.

Cardiovascular Endurance

Cardiovascular training is another fitness component that needs to be considered when training for birth. Interval training most closely resembles the demands of birth itself, and it should play a role in your pregnancy cardio training. Low-impact activities that will elevate the heart rate are the best choices because they will improve cardiovascular fitness while protecting the pelvic floor from additional strain. If you are a runner or if you participate in activities with a lot of jumping or in other impact activities, you may wish to adjust your training to find low-or no-impact exercises. While running and jumping are perfectly safe, they do place the already compromised core under additional strain that is perhaps not optimal. Changes in the center of gravity and hormonal influences that increase mobility and instability of the pelvis are reasons to seek out alternatives to running and jumping in pregnancy. Activities like walking (especially hill walking), swimming, and elliptical training are great choices. Spinning and cycling may be options as well, but pay attention to your pelvic alignment, your body temperature (you don't want to overheat), and your rate of perceived exertion.

Stretch and Release Work

An often overlooked aspect of training is stretch and release work. Flexible, supple muscles are better able to release and yield as they need to during birth. Tight (also called hypertonic), overused muscles will restrict the space in the pelvis, resist the need to release, and be more likely to become injured during birth. As with any muscle in the body, the balance between strength and length is important. Stretch and release work that targets the muscles in the pelvic floor, the adductors, the glutes, and the hip flexors is a great way to optimize the pelvis in pregnancy and ensure it can respond to the needs of labor in a positive way. We will cover this in more detail in chapter 3.

Functional Movement for Motherhood

As a mom caring for babies and children, you will move your body in ways that you may rarely or never have done before. The most common movements for motherhood are squatting, lifting, carrying, pushing, pulling, rotating, bending, and balancing. Daily life will include lifting and carrying your baby, lifting and carrying a car seat (with and without your baby), bending and lifting your baby out of the crib, and rotating in the car to check on your child in the car seat. You will bend and squat and lift doing the many loads of laundry that are required—you will be busy! Ideally, you will start doing these moves after the first few weeks of recovery because rest is critical. You should not be doing loads of laundry or carrying your baby in a car seat right after your baby is born. Delegate those tasks to your doula or family so you can focus on resting and healing and then gradually start to bring movement into your day. Remember, there is movement and there is exercise. As a busy mom, you will be getting a lot of movement. Women who are concerned that they are too busy to make it to the gym for their workouts or do any exercise at home should not discount that their busy lives are full of movement. Besides, the early weeks postpartum are meant for rest, healing, and recovery. Restorative exercises (such as those you will learn in chapter 14) and gradual daily motherhood movements are all you need to worry about, and learning them while still pregnant will make the recovery and core restoration much easier!

Take Action

Squatting is a movement that as children we do perfectly all day. As we grow up, we start to bend as opposed to squat and, while both movements are natural, squatting ends up being replaced by other movements. Squatting is a fantastic position for labor and is the movement we should use to pick things up off the floor, but because adults do less squatting, women are not prepared for using it in labor. Practice squats as part of your daily movement, make them a focus in your workouts, and try to transition to squatting for elimination (bowel movements). You can put some small stools (no pun intended) at the base of your toilet or try the squatty potty – a stool that wraps around the base of your toilet. This elevates the knees so they are above the pelvis, as in a squat, and allows the puborectalis muscle (a muscle that loops around the rectum) to relax so stool can come out faster and easier. By adding squats to your daily routine, you will build a better birthing body and be ready to use this amazing position in your labor.

Squatting has been shown to increase the pelvic diameter. This means there is more space in the pelvis and more space is good when we want to facilitate birth. A 1982 study by Russell indicated that squatting increases the pelvic outlet by one centimeter in the transverse diameter (side to side) and two centimeters in the antero-posterior diameter (front to back). The overall result is an increase of 28 percent in area compared with the lithotomy (lying on the back) position (Russell 1982). While this is an older study, the findings still ring true today. This sounds great, but if you haven't been accustomed to squatting and then try to do it in labor, you may not find the success you were hoping for. This is usually because those who don't squat regularly have tightness in parts of the legs that prevent the squat from being performed correctly.

Squatting in labor is best done with the feet parallel and the knees pointing forward. This keeps the most space between the sitting bones, which is what we want for birth. A well-executed squat in pregnancy, therefore, is best practiced with the feet as parallel and pointing forward as is comfortable for you (see figure 2.1a). Most people who are not used to squatting will perform it with the feet and knees pointing outward (see figure 2.1b). This actually reduces the space in the pelvis, which is the opposite of what you want. Practice squatting daily and work in a comfortable range of motion that allows you to squat correctly: with your knees and feet pointing forward and where you can keep your tailbone from tucking underneath you.

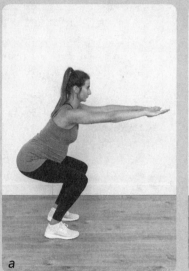
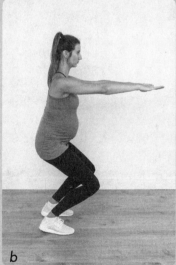

Figure 2.1   Squat: (a) correct and (b) incorrect.

FULL-BODY FITNESS THROUGH THE TRIMESTERS

Now we are going to take a detailed look at exercising through the trimesters. Later chapters will dive deeper into the actual exercises as well as specific programs to keep you fit at every stage. This section is meant to touch on the key points to consider as well as introduce the concept of a fourth trimester, which comprises the first three months postpartum.

First Trimester

As mentioned, movement in the first trimester can be a struggle due to decreased energy levels and the onset of nausea. If you are finding it hard to do anything other than survive, don't panic. It will pass. When you can, go for a walk and if that is all you can do—awesome! If your energy allows you more freedom for movement in your day, always take the time for a walk, ideally in minimal shoes (more on this later). For your strength, cardio, and release work, focus on connecting with your pelvic floor and deep core. You'll want to do one to two minutes of core breathing on its own daily (you will learn this exercise in chapter 6) and add it to moves like the clam shell, squats, and even biceps curls to turn any exercise into a core exercise. Moves like clam shells where you're in a side-lying position (you will learn this exercise in chapter 7) and squats are great for building strength and endurance in the glutes and legs as well as being fantastic birth preparation exercises. Having a body that is accustomed to the movements used in labor and birth *before* the big day arrives will ensure you are ready to not only handle the challenge but perform really well!

Take Action

Parents-to-be usually wait to purchase an infant car seat until close to the due date, but we recommend that you buy it as early in your pregnancy as possible so you can use it in your training. Kettlebells and dumbbells work as substitutes, but why not train with the exact thing that you will be lifting over and over again? Remember, be as specific as possible in your training to get your body ready for real life. A car seat is awkward and heavy (and becomes heavier once your baby is in it and as your baby grows!). Practice lifting your car seat, carrying it, transferring it into and out of the car, and swinging it gently to soothe your baby. These are all things you will do with it once your baby has arrived. Finally, be sure to practice holding it and walking with it in one hand and then the other hand, so you keep your muscles balanced and are able to use either hand as the situation requires.

Second Trimester

The second trimester typically brings renewed vigor. Nausea has usually passed by now, energy levels are higher, and even though you will be showing, your belly will not really limit you in your movement. Higher repetitions, more sets, and new exercises are available to you, but still make sure you take time to relax, unwind, stretch, and release. A daily walk remains a priority as well. Add in some hills or some stairs for low-impact cardio that gets your heart rate up while respecting your pelvic floor. Exercising in the supine position (lying on your back) is typically not advised; this is due to the potential of compressing the inferior vena cava (a large vein that carries blood from the lower body back to the heart). This compression can lead to dizziness, a drop in blood pressure, and fluid retention. Some women do fine lying on their backs even late into the pregnancy, while others need to use pillows or bolsters so their head is higher than their hips for supine floor work.

Third Trimester

The third trimester is the home stretch. You have three months left to really prepare your body for labor and birth. In the first month or so, your energy should still be adequate, but in months eight and nine, you will most likely start to feel like slowing down, nesting, and starting to count down the days. Slowing down is a good thing and is essential—think of it like tapering before a big race. You have done the training and the prep work and race day is not far away. As you continue your workouts, you will naturally begin to back off the reps and the weight and opt for lighter workouts that will allow you to keep some energy in the tank for the big day. Focus on lots of release work for the pelvic floor and surrounding muscles like the glutes, inner thighs, and hamstrings. Using a stability ball pressed against a wall behind you while you hold a deep squat position can be a nice way

BODY FACT

During pregnancy the heart works very efficiently and will eject more blood per beat. By the second trimester your heart at rest will be working about 40 percent harder than it was when you weren't pregnant. Your blood volume also increases progressively during pregnancy, beginning in weeks six to eight and continuing until weeks 32 to 34. The volume of plasma increases by about 40 percent to 50 percent, and red blood cell mass increases by about 20 percent to 30 percent. This greater blood volume and circulation rate then creates the need for increased iron and folic acid intake.

to build endurance in your legs while also creating some space and stretch in the pelvic floor. Thinking about the most optimal birthing positions and then practicing them daily is key. Side-lying positions, supported squat positions, tall kneeling positions, and positions on all fours are considered great choices when it comes to labor and birth. In later chapters, we are going to show you exercises that mimic these positions and will help you build an amazing body for birth!

Moving during early labor will help you better manage the discomfort, facilitate the passage for your baby, and allow the muscles in the core to be able to help with the process. Walking is a convenient and helpful movement, and since you will have been doing it every day of your pregnancy you will have the energy and stamina available for this in your labor. When it comes time to transition to the second stage of labor, the pushing phase, it is ideal to position yourself so that gravity can assist you. Also, you want to ensure your sacrum stays free so it can move as the baby moves. The common back-lying or lithotomy position can actually work against the birthing process because gravity is taken out of the picture. Furthermore, the bed pushing against the sacrum limits the space in the pelvis and prevents the natural movement of the sacrum as baby moves into the vaginal canal. Ideally, chose an alternative like side-lying, supported squatting, staggered standing, or all fours. The side-lying position has been shown to offer a protective element to the perineum and the pelvic floor, and it can be helpful if you have a labor that is progressing very quickly and you would like to slow things down. All-fours positions such as kneeling on the hospital bed or draping yourself over a ball are lovely supportive positions that utilize gravity and keep the sacrum free. Staggered standing with one leg elevated on a stool or chair uses gravity and keeps the sacrum free while the asymmetry in the pelvis can often help the baby navigate through the pelvis. The key is variety and movement. One position may work for a while and then you may need to switch things up and come back to the original position later. Stay fluid and trust that your movement is helping facilitate the process.

Fourth Trimester

The fourth trimester is the recovery phase and is absolutely essential to regaining core function. The focus is on rest, recovery, and core retraining. Too many women jump immediately into training and leave out the element of retraining, only to face challenges such as lingering back pain, a tummy that won't lie flat, and even things like incontinence and other forms of pelvic floor dysfunction.

After your baby is born, regardless of whether you had a vaginal birth or a cesarean birth, you need time to recover. Ensure you have support from a doula or your family during the first few weeks so you can focus on rest and healing your postpartum body. Ice packs for your perineum are soothing for the first 24 hours (you can freeze sanitary pads or you can purchase soft gel ice packs). Following the first day, heat in the form of sitz baths multiple times a day will help. Belly wrapping is used in many cultures around the world and is slowly gaining traction in North America. Not to be confused with waist training, the gentle practice of belly wrapping provides external support to the tissues in the pelvis and abdominal wall while they heal. It is important to couple a belly wrap with restorative exercise and ensure the wrap is put on from the bottom up to take pressure off the healing pelvic floor.

The pressure placed on new moms to "get their bodies back" is immense; however, it needs to be ignored. After performing one of the most incredible feats of physical and mental strength, many new moms unfortunately don't meet their own standards and feel weak and out of shape. They are therefore vulnerable to the claims of exercise classes promoting quick results and are looking for the hardest, most intense activity that will help them feel strong again. Keep in mind, your body has just been through nine months of changes and adaptations that culminated in the birth of your baby. It is not realistic to expect your body to just bounce back to the way it was before pregnancy. The truth is, your body has changed and it will never be the same. That is not to say it can't be better, stronger, or more functional, but it will never be the same as it was and striving to get back to what it was is futile. Instead, your focus should be on retraining your core and then gradually progressing back to more intense activities. Fitness choices such as boot camp or running are things that you may return to once your core is restored but they are not the activities to choose in an attempt to "get your body back."

The first six to eight weeks postpartum are meant for rest and recovery with gentle core restoration work added at a gradual pace. A pelvic floor physiotherapy assessment around six weeks postpartum is recommended for every woman regardless of how you gave birth. This is an overlooked aspect of women's health that should be the standard of care and a mandatory piece of prenatal and postpartum healthcare. The traditional belief is that at six weeks postpartum women can get the green light to go back to regular activities. Currently, women take this as a thumbs up to start running or get back to the CrossFit box. The postpartum body is simply not ready for the demands of activities like running and full scale CrossFit at six weeks postpartum and may not be until around four, six, or even 12 months postpartum. Your pelvic floor physiotherapist is an essential part of your health care team and should be the one to give you the green light for a return to more intense activities. This is an escape from current norms, but as word gets out about the importance of pelvic health, more and more women are choosing to be proactive in their pregnancies and are honoring the need to recover. The hopes are that the increasing rates of incontinence and pelvic organ prolapse will start to retreat and we will see women feeling strong and confident in their postpartum bodies instead of feeling weak and broken.

Take Action

You may have read about creating a birth plan, which we think is a great idea. But we would also recommend you create a recovery plan as well. Recovery is just as important as the birth, and preparing ahead of time is key. Think about such things as ice packs, healing herbs for your perineum, premade meals, an abdominal wrap, booking a pelvic floor physiotherapy appointment for six to eight weeks after your due date, and knowing who is on your postpartum support team—family members, friends, maybe even a postpartum doula. And one final thing: think of your birth plan more like a birth guide. Birth is a very dynamic, organic process and not everything goes as planned. Be sure to keep an open mind, have a guide to refer to, and build a strong birth team to help support you through it.

Training for a big event requires deliberate, intentional movement that prepares the body to perform, reduces the chances of injury, and primes the body to heal once the event is completed. Training for birth is no different. This book is increasing your knowledge about the changes that are happening and how you can best support your body through these changes and build an incredible birthing body. The next chapters will delve deeper into the core—namely, the pelvic floor, diaphragm, and abdomen—which perhaps undergoes the most significant of all the changes in pregnancy and birth.

3

The Pelvic Floor: The Foundation of the Core

The pelvic floor is a part of the body that doesn't get a lot of attention, but during pregnancy you're likely to start thinking about it and wondering how to prepare the area for your baby's birth. You may have heard about Kegels or been told to do them, but there is so much more you can do to prepare. This chapter will give you information you won't believe you haven't heard before!

WHAT IS THE PELVIC FLOOR?

The pelvic floor is the foundation of the Core 4, the group of deep muscles we introduced in the last chapter that are responsible for stabilizing and helping control your body's movement. Together with the diaphragm, transversus abdominis, and multifidus, the pelvic floor has a role in breathing, creating tension in your abdominal wall, and stabilizing your spine and pelvis (see figure 3.1).

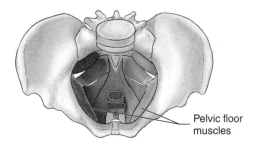

Pelvic floor muscles

Figure 3.1   The pelvic floor.

The pelvic floor is a collection of muscles, nerves, tendons, blood vessels, ligaments, and connective tissue all interwoven in your pelvis. It attaches to your pubic bone (which is actually a joint but for simplicity we will say bone) in front, to your tailbone (coccyx) in back, and to your sitz bones (ischial tuberosities) on each side. It forms the base of the pelvis and has many important functions such as being responsible for sexual response and continence. It is astonishing that for a part of our body that does so much, we generally know so little about it. Unfortunately, it is not until there is a problem in the pelvis that women are given the information they should have been told before.

Pelvic Floor Function

As the foundation of the core, the pelvic floor helps support the pelvic organs: bladder, rectum, and your growing uterus (see figure 3.2). It also plays a role in urinary continence so you can control when you eliminate and don't pee when you cough, run, or jump. The pelvic floor muscles also stabilize your spine and pelvis as mentioned in the previous chapter. During birth, the pelvic floor muscles must yield to allow baby to pass through the birth canal, and there is an ejection reflex that will help to push your baby out. For all this to occur, often all at once, the pelvic floor muscles must have strength, endurance, timing, coordination, and control. Kegel exercises (voluntary pelvic floor contractions followed by relaxation) can help, but they are not for everyone, because many women do them incorrectly. Kegels also reflect a limited view of the abilities of the pelvic floor.

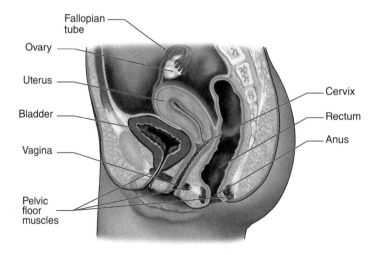

Figure 3.2   The pelvic floor and the supported organs.

What Is a Pelvic Floor Physiotherapist?

Pelvic floor physiotherapy is the most underused service in women's health, and many women don't even know it exists until they have a problem to fix. Pelvic floor physiotherapists are first trained to perform general physiotherapy and then take additional training that addresses the pelvic floor. They perform internal (vaginal and rectal) assessments to determine the function of the muscles and position of the organs, to mobilize any scar tissue, and to teach women how to properly contract and relax their pelvic floor. They help balance the pelvis to ensure the pelvic muscles are aligned and able to do their job, they help release unproductive tension patterns that may interfere with labor and birth, and they help women identify the right and wrong way to engage the pelvic floor. Many pelvic floor physiotherapists have additional training to help women understand what their body needs to do when they are pushing their baby out. These therapists are also an essential part of your prenatal health care team and your postpartum recovery, and all new moms should see one around six weeks postpartum. In fact, as mentioned in the last chapter, you should rely on your pelvic floor physiotherapist to give you the green light to return to high-impact activities (and it will not be at six weeks postpartum!).

Because it is a part of the body that is vital to so many aspects of our daily life, and also because it is a part of the body we can't see, it is important to have a therapist who can help us access and optimize it.

Kegels are in essence an isolated exercise, yet given that we are dynamic beings who move throughout the day (at least ideally), it makes sense to broaden the view of pelvic floor exercise to include movement. It's all well and good to know how to isolate your pelvic floor muscles, but because they work in synergy with the Core 4 as the foundation to all movement, it is important to integrate the pelvic floor muscles into functional movements of daily living. Chapter 9 has been dedicated to this aim with Movement for Motherhood, which will teach you how to use your pelvic floor and Core 4 in a variety of daily movements and activities.

In addition to supporting movement, the pelvic floor muscles have a role in breathing and controlling intra-abdominal pressure and therefore must work synergistically with the diaphragm, the transversus abdominis, and the multifidus, making up the Core 4 as mentioned earlier. The Core 4 form the deepest layer of the core and work together to ensure alignment, proper biomechanics, and control during activities. They are anticipatory, meaning they prepare us for movement and they also stabilize and control movement.

Take Action

To do a proper Kegel, sit on an exercise ball or a firm chair. You can place your hand under your perineum to give more feedback or simply allow the roundness of the ball to give you the feedback. Be sure you are in good alignment by sitting on your sitz bones and feeling your perineum on the surface of the ball or chair. Now, take a breath in and as you exhale, imagine picking up a blueberry with your vagina and drawing it up and into your body. As you inhale, lower it down again. Did you feel your perineum lift up off the ball? Be sure not to "squeeze" the blueberry; the goal is not to make blueberry juice. It is the "lift" that is critical to the proper use of the pelvic floor muscles. And be sure not to try too hard— you are not picking up pianos here, just a tiny little blueberry, so use a firm but gentle grip and lift followed by a letting go. We like to also use a term called the "core breath" to help instill the importance of the breath working in coordination with the pelvic floor and overall core. We go into more detail about this in the next chapter.

If you are comfortable inserting a finger into your vagina while you do the Core Breath (Kegel), you will feel a gentle squeeze and lift, or drawing up and into your body. Then you should feel the lowering down again as you release. You can also ask your partner to insert a finger or penis and test this way. Many women test on the toilet by trying to stop the flow of urine; however, this is not recommended because it can confuse the bladder and is only testing the squeeze component of the exercise, which you actually want to deemphasize.

Because the pelvic floor muscles are engaged in anticipation of most movement, you will in fact be exercising your pelvic floor every time you rise out of a chair, lift your arm, pick something up, or step forward.

Adding intentional breathing and cues like the blueberry to a Kegel enhances the synergy of the Core 4. This type of breathing is called the core breath, which you will learn more about in the next chapter.

The diaphragm, as shown in figure 3.3, is the largest muscle used for breathing. The diaphragm is located in the ribcage and attaches into the lumbar spine. It is a dome shape at rest and becomes flatter in shape as you breathe in. This movement forces the ribs to move out to the side.

Unfortunately, many people actually use this muscle incorrectly. Each breath should be accompanied by lateral rib expansion, yet with today's sedentary lifestyle and slouched posture many people tend to breathe up in the chest. This has a major impact on the synergy with the pelvic floor. When you breathe in, the diaphragm should contract and descend and the pelvic floor should then lengthen and descend. The transversus abdominis

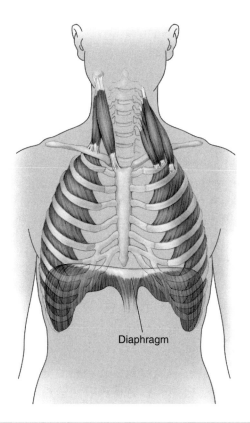

Figure 3.3   The diaphragm.

should also lengthen and expand outward to allow the air to enter the body freely. When you exhale the opposite happens—the pelvic floor contracts and lifts, the transversus moves inward, and the diaphragm rises up. To help you master this synergy you will learn and practice the core breath, a fundamental exercise to practice daily in pregnancy to help minimize things like diastasis and back pain. The core breath is a key exercise for postpartum recovery as well.

Pelvic Floor Dysfunction

Pregnancy and birth are often blamed for many of the core challenges women face postpartum. Common struggles include incontinence, pelvic organ prolapse, pelvic pain, lower-back pain, and a tummy that simply won't lie flat anymore. Women have a false belief that because they have had children, it is normal to have these challenges. This is not true. It is not normal—common, but not normal—and so much of what women deal with postpartum can be prevented or minimized if they are given the right information during pregnancy.

The old standard for treating pelvic floor dysfunction was for the OBGYN to dole out a standardized sheet of Kegel exercises. Science and clinical experience shows us that this is not only ineffective but can be harmful to some women. The three personalities of the pelvic floor demonstrate why certain women should not necessarily do Kegels. Most of us envision that after a baby's ten-centimeter head comes through our vagina, the vagina will be left stretched and weak; hence, there is a need for Kegels. This is true in many cases postpartum, if the pelvic floor has been stretched and has not yet recovered its normal tone, strength, endurance, and timing. You can think of this pelvic floor as the "beach bum." The tissue is long and lax (hypotonic) and not really working very well. Untreated, most women with this type of pelvic floor will develop incontinence, prolapse, and perhaps pain. Kegels can and should help these women, especially when used during movement. However, there is another personality of the pelvic floor we call the "gym rat." This pelvic floor is tight (hypertonic), contracted, and can be short; therefore, it also has no power and poor timing. With this type of pelvic floor, women still have incontinence. Often, they will have pelvic pain, especially pain during intercourse. This pelvic floor has no give, and doing Kegels will worsen any dysfunction because the Kegels will be contracting an already contracted group of muscles. The third personality of the pelvic floor, "the little gymnast," is what we should all strive for, where there is a perfect balance of tone, flexibility, and timing. This is a floor that can support a pregnancy, stretch for birth, and return to optimal Core 4 synergy.

As we have discussed, our bodies are amazing at compensating. The pelvic floor muscles often come to the rescue and attempt to do the work of the abdominals that are now stretched and weakened and therefore ineffective. This most often results in pelvic floor muscles that are hypertonic and short, disrupting the synergy of the Core 4. Having Core 4 muscles that are not in sync will contribute to pelvic floor dysfunction such as urinary incontinence, pelvic organ prolapse, and pelvic pain. It is often thought that these conditions only happen to older women, but pelvic floor dysfunction can affect women at any age and any stage of life. You may have heard of your grandmother or aunt having pelvic organ prolapse, or your friends leaking pee when they exercise ever since they had kids. These issues are common but they are not normal, and in pregnancy there is a lot you can do to avoid these conditions.

Your postpartum recovery is key as well. It is a time of healing, restoration, and retraining. The pelvic floor will have been through a lot, and getting started with core breathing as soon as possible postpartum will go a long way to restoring form and function and avoiding dysfunctions. Let's take a closer look at these common dysfunctions.

Urinary Incontinence

By definition, incontinence is any unwanted loss of urine at any time and of any amount. You may hear women say that it is normal to leak after having kids, but the truth is it is *not* normal.

There are two main types of incontinence: stress urinary incontinence (SUI) and urge urinary incontinence (UUI). SUI occurs when there is an increase in intra-abdominal pressure that is too great for the sphincters and pelvic floor to manage. Small amounts of urine leak out with exertion such as laughing, coughing, sneezing, and running. UUI typically involves a sudden, often uncontrollable, need to find a bathroom. It can be the result of nerve damage or scar tissue, or it can even be behavioral. It is also possible to have both types; this is called mixed incontinence.

During pregnancy the need to urinate can increase under the effects of hormones and the pressure on the bladder as baby grows. It is also common to experience some form of incontinence as well. Studies show that if you experience incontinence in your pregnancy, there is a 70 percent chance that you will continue to live with it postpartum as well (Rocha, Brandao, Melo, Torres, Mota, and Costa 2017).

Pelvic Organ Prolapse

Pelvic organ prolapse is the descent of the pelvic organs (bladder, uterus, or rectum) into the vaginal canal. A cystocele occurs when the bladder bulges into the vaginal wall (also called an anterior wall prolapse). A uterine prolapse occurs when the uterus starts to descend into the vagina. A rectocele is when the rectum bulges into the vagina (also called a posterior wall prolapse). There are varying degrees of prolapse ranging from grade 1, which is very mild, to grade 4, which most often requires surgery. An important thing to note about prolapse is that the degree of descent doesn't necessarily correlate with the symptoms. Some women may have a small prolapse and be very symptomatic, while others will have a more advanced prolapse yet have no symptoms at all.

Some common signs of prolapse may be lower-back pain, a sense of heaviness in the pelvis, a tugging or pulling sensation, a feeling like something is falling out, pain with intercourse, inability to insert a tampon, or

BODY FACT

The pudendal nerve is the main nerve of the perineum. It is a sensory, autonomic, and motor nerve that carries signals to and from the anus, the genitals, and the urethra. It is a nerve that can be injured in childbirth due to stretch, compression, or cutting from an episiotomy. Injury to the pudendal nerve can contribute to incontinence, prolapse, and chronic pain conditions.

inability to keep a tampon in. These are just a few of the symptoms, and they are felt to different degrees by different women. Like we said, some may feel symptoms when they have an early stage prolapse while others feel nothing at all and only notice the prolapse once there is a bulge at the entrance to the vagina.

Pelvic organ prolapse is not life threatening, but it is life altering. Especially for active women, it can be a very unpleasant reality. Also note that prolapse can take years to develop and, because not everyone feels the early signs and symptoms, it is important to seek out a pelvic floor physiotherapist as part of your health care team in pregnancy and for the rest of your life. If you do not have access to a qualified pelvic floor physiotherapist and you suspect you have a prolapse, accessing resources online like the Association for Pelvic Organ Prolapse Support (APOPS) and asking your OBGYN to do a POP-Q (a special test to measure the grade of prolapse) can help you make informed choices about your health care. Posture, alignment, proper body mechanics, Core 4 synergy, preparing your body for birth, recovering optimally, and delaying the return to high-impact activities will all play a role in preventing or minimizing the descent of the pelvic organs.

Pelvic Pain

Pelvic pain is another dysfunction often brushed off as just another pregnancy ailment. However, just because you are pregnant does not mean you need to suffer. Things like lower-back pain, sacroiliac joint pain, pubic symphysis diastasis (pain in the front of your pelvis at the pubic joint), and dyspareunia (pain during sex) can all be treated and often cured during pregnancy or postpartum. Often the problem is as simple as the pelvic floor muscles being hypertonic (too tight), or hypotonic (too lax). Other problems include compensatory strategies coming into play, such as referred pain from other muscles like the hip adductors, or uneven rotational forces on the pelvic bones. Once again, posture, alignment, and synergy in the Core 4 play important roles in prevention and treatment of pelvic floor dysfunctions during pregnancy.

BODY FACT

When the pelvis is in a neutral position, with the sitz bones rooted down toward the ground and the pubic joint and the two hip bones in the same plane, the bladder receives bony support from the pubic joint. When the pelvis is posteriorly tilted, this bony support is lost and the bladder loses an element of support. A posteriorly tilted pelvis can also place undue strain on the ligament that attaches from the sacrum to the uterus—the uterosacral ligament—and can potentially contribute to uterine prolapse.

PREGNANCY AND BIRTH'S IMPACT ON THE PELVIC FLOOR

The pelvic floor undergoes tremendous change and adaptation in pregnancy and birth. Hormones are making the joints in the pelvis more mobile, which requires the pelvic floor to work a little harder to maintain stability and control. This results in compensations— other muscles being called upon to help compensate for the changes in the pelvic floor. This in turn affects the synergy, or the coordination and timing, of the Core 4. In the short term, compensations are helpful, but over time they lead to dyssynergy and dysfunction in the pelvic floor.

As the baby grows, so does the uterus. The need to support this ever-increasing weight not only places strain on the pelvic floor directly but also challenges your posture. As your belly grows and you adjust your alignment to counter the weight, the pelvis tips and forces the pelvic floor into less-than-optimal positions.

One of the greatest challenges to the pelvic floor is birth. During vaginal birth, as the baby descends there is potential for injury to the tissues in the vaginal canal, the nerves, the pelvic floor, and the perineum. The soft tissues are prone to tearing, the nerves can be compressed or stretched, and, in some cases, pelvic bones can be fractured. The pushing phase will often see a massive increase in intra-abdominal pressure against the pelvic organs. Thinking back to the fact that hormones increase the laxity of the pelvic floor structures and ligaments, we can see how directed Valsalva pushing, otherwise known as purple pushing, can overstretch the ligaments and contribute to prolapse.

Many believe that the pelvic floor is spared during a cesarean birth; however, this is not the case. Women who have cesareans also have the same hormonal influences, the same postural changes, the same alignment shifts, and the same additional weight on the pelvic floor. In addition to the same pregnancy challenges, most women still go through the pushing phase for some time once the cervix is dilated and then end up giving birth via cesarean. Other women even have some early success with pushing but then experience "failure to progress" or "stalled labor," resulting in an unplanned cesarean. But, even with a planned cesarean birth, there are consequences to the pelvic floor.

BODY FACT

The weight and size of the uterus changes a lot in pregnancy. It goes from weighing roughly 2 ounces (50 g; about the size of a small orange) to about 2 pounds (1 kg; the size of a watermelon!). After the baby is born the process of the uterus returning to its nonpregnant state is called involution.

PREVENTING PELVIC FLOOR DYSFUNCTION

Pregnancy is an ideal time to learn about and train the pelvic floor. It will undergo considerable changes in pregnancy and face significant challenges during birth, so you want to make sure it is optimized and ready to handle whatever labor and birth bring its way. It is also important to know how to best heal your pelvic floor once your baby is born.

The current trend in pregnancy fitness is for women to lift really heavy weights while pregnant and then return to high-intensity training mere weeks after the baby is born. Extremes in pregnancy are applauded, and many women are now pursuing or continuing high-intensity activities during their pregnancy. While we certainly believe that women can and should move, lift, pull, carry, twist, and bend, we don't believe that it should be done at the intensity that is currently the trend. While pregnancy shouldn't stop you from being active, we recommend that you modify certain activities so that your pelvic floor and core are not forced to deal with more than they already are. We also don't believe that harder, faster, heavier is the way to recover, either. Too many times we have seen women jump back into fitness far too soon with a body that simply was not ready, only to regret the decision and be faced with pelvic floor dysfunction that required major modifications to their movement lifestyle.

Slow, steady, and gradual progression is what the body needs to recover. It took nine months to grow a person, followed by the demands of birth. It is not realistic to think that the body, especially the pelvic floor, is ready for intense activity such as bouncing, jumping, or heavy lifting in the early months postpartum. In reality, it will take between 4 to 12 months to truly be ready to return to the higher-impact activities like boot camp, CrossFit, or running. Start with low-impact activities like squats, lunges, walking,

BODY FACT

An episiotomy is a surgical cut of the perineum made during delivery. It is a cut through the skin, the transverse perineal muscle, the bulbocavernosus muscle, and the vaginal wall (epithelium). It used to be standard practice to perform an episiotomy on every birthing woman. It was thought that creating more space would facilitate the birth. Over time, it was determined that episiotomies actually encouraged more severe perineal injuries, so they are no longer routinely performed. Be sure to ask your care provider if they perform routine episiotomies. Ideally, your healthcare provider will use an episiotomy only in an urgent emergency situation.

cycling, and swimming. Scale back the intensity of your favorite classes as you start to reintegrate impact movements. As you retrain your system, your strength and endurance will return, and when your body is ready, you will be able to resume training with higher-impact activities.

Scaling down and choosing low-or no-impact activities in your pregnancy can go a long way to preserving the integrity of your pelvic floor. Training during pregnancy is less about reaching distance goals or weight goals, and more about readying your body for one of the most challenging events you will ever do. Taking steps to modify your exercise routine as your pregnancy progresses and rebuilding your fitness with retraining movement postpartum is your best insurance policy to prevent pelvic floor dysfunction. Working with this preventive mindset will set you up for a more comfortable pregnancy, a better birth, and a smoother transition to motherhood! Here are some proven strategies to follow to prevent pelvic floor dysfunction.

Maintain Proper Posture and Alignment

Posture and alignment are key to prevention. Keeping the pelvis in a neutral position, keeping the ribs stacked over the pelvis, and ensuring your day has a lot of natural movement like walking and squatting will help. When we sit, we often sit with a tucked-under tailbone or on our sacrum. Most of the chairs we use set us up for a posteriorly tilted pelvis and that needs to change. But until we get better chairs and sit less, pay attention to your sitting posture. Sit on your sitz bones, not on your sacrum. Constantly sitting with a tucked-under tailbone can shorten and tighten the pelvic floor (this is not ideal for birth) and puts an unnatural load on the uterosacral ligament (not great for your uterus). It is also problematic for your spine because it changes the natural lordotic curve and compromises the discs. Ideally, you should sit less often. When you do have to sit, vary your position, find a neutral pelvis and don't sit for extended periods. Take many movement breaks throughout your day and consider trying a standing desk.

Wear Minimal Shoes

It is advisable to wear minimal (flat) shoes as much as possible, especially while standing and moving. This may sound strange, but wearing heels pitches you forward and you certainly don't need more of that when your pregnant belly is already stressing your alignment. When your weight combined with the heels is pitching you forward, the tendency is to then lean back and tuck the pelvis. As we mentioned above, that is not ideal, so ditch the heels and opt for flat, minimal shoes. This will also help keep your calves and hamstrings lengthened.

Stretch the Calves and Hamstrings Daily

While minimal shoes, as mentioned previously, are helpful, daily calf and hamstring stretching will also help the pelvis find and stay in a neutral position. When the backs of your legs are tight (often from too much sitting and wearing heeled shoes) it pulls the pelvis posteriorly—again, not ideal for the pelvic floor. In chapter 5 you will learn some great release techniques to stretch your calves and hamstrings.

Learn How to Do Kegel Exercises

Kegels, also known as pelvic floor muscle exercises, are becoming more mainstream thanks to social media. The benefits of doing Kegels are well documented both in prevention and recovery from injury, incontinence, and prolapse. However, studies also show that most women do them incorrectly if at all. The gold standard for determining whether you are doing Kegels correctly is having an internal assessment by a pelvic floor physiotherapist, who will be able to tell you if you are contracting correctly, and, just as important, if you are releasing correctly. If this assessment is not available to you, refer back to earlier in the chapter where we discussed how to do a Kegel. Also, remember the three personalities of the pelvic floor—hypotonic, hypertonic, and the little gymnast (just right)—because it is important to know if and when Kegels are appropriate for you.

Use Core Breathing

The core breath is a more comprehensive approach to Kegels. It may be a better option for you because it ties in breathing with engagement of the pelvic floor. In the later stages of pregnancy, learning how to use the core breath and the pelvic floor to push the baby out while minimizing intra-abdominal pressure can help minimize some of the negative effects of birth on the pelvic floor. Again, you will learn more about how the core breath relates to the abdominals in chapter 4 and a step-by-step exercise in chapter 6.

Prepare to Push

Using different positions during labor, especially during the pushing phase, can help prevent the common injuries sustained during birth. Upright, gravity-assisted positions such as those mentioned in chapter 2 can help shorten the labor phase. Side-lying and all-fours positions have been shown to reduce tearing in your perineum as compared to back-lying and semi-recumbent birthing positions. Practicing getting into and out of these positions during your pregnancy will make the transitions easier during labor and birth. Take it one step further and practice releasing your pelvic floor to open the pelvic door in these positions. The more comfortable you feel in these positions the easier they are to use and the more effective your pushing will be, thereby minimizing exhaustion, failure to progress, and the use of interventions.

Massage Your Perineum

Perineal massage is a great practice and has many benefits. It can increase blood flow to the area and help increase the viscoelasticity of your pelvic floor, thereby helping to prevent tearing. Also, it can help break down any adhesions from previous births, trauma, or compensations. Third, and perhaps most important, it will help you learn to yield to the discomfort of birth rather than tensing up. Ultimately, perineal massage is meant to give you an opportunity to feel pressure and discomfort in the area in order to train your pelvic floor (and brain) to respond appropriately by releasing tension in the presence of discomfort, which closely mimics the crowning phase of labor when your baby is emerging into the world. The massage is typically done starting around week 36 and can be done by yourself or by your partner. We explain the method in detail in chapter 5.

Take Action

The pelvic floor muscles need strength, coordination, control, endurance, and timing. You can improve all of these with different types of exercises. Try these two "fancy" Kegels.

Stairs

This exercise builds endurance, normal tone, strength, coordination, and control. This is different from a regular Kegel because it has you contract on a four count and release on a four count. This one is quite useful for treating prolapse. Think of it as if you are going up imaginary stairs with your pelvic floor muscles.

To perform the exercise, sit or stand in proper posture and imagine picking up a blueberry with your vagina and drawing it up and into your body. As you draw the blueberry up and in, pause at floor 1 (one-fourth of the way up), then contract and lift again to get to floor 2 (you are now halfway up). Resume contracting and lifting to get to floor 3, and finally contract and lift the blueberry to floor 4, at the top of your vagina. Once at the top, pause and then slowly release to lower back down to floor 3, pause and continue to release down to floor 2, then to floor 1, and finally back down to full release.

Locking or Knack

This is a very popular pelvic floor muscle training exercise because it works on timing, therefore helping to cure incontinence. It is essential to regain the timing of the pelvic floor when faced with increases in intra-abdominal pressure. For this exercise, you will pick up your blueberry and lower it down as fast as you can as long as you can get a perfect lift all the way to the fourth floor (see the previous exercise, "Stairs").

To perform this exercise, sit or stand in good alignment and imagine picking up your blueberry with your vagina and drawing it up and in as fast as you can. Release the blueberry back down as fast as you can and repeat for as many as you can do perfectly. Once you lose form or can't reach the fourth floor, you are done. Start slow if you need to. The Knack incorporates this exercise into daily life as a precontraction before coughing or sneezing. Quality with pelvic floor muscle training is more important than quantity.

The pelvic floor is the foundation of the core, working tirelessly to support and stabilize your pelvis and spine. Together with the diaphragm, multifidus, and transversus abdominis, it forms the Core 4. In the next chapter, we will take a closer look at the abdominals and how they are affected by pregnancy.

The Abdominals: During Pregnancy and Beyond

4

As discussed in previous chapters, pregnancy causes many changes throughout the body, but it is the "bump" that gets all the attention. The abdominal wall is lovingly referred to as the baby bump or the belly in pregnancy and is the center of attention in pregnancy photos. After the baby is born however, it becomes an area of the body that is unappreciated, hidden, and sometimes even loathed.

The ultimate goal for most new moms is to lose their tummies and get their bodies back. Unfortunately, many new moms will go on diets and start intense workouts too soon postpartum. In an attempt to flatten their abs, they choose the most aggressive core exercises, overlooking the need to rest, recover, and retrain the core first. But with the right information, you can help maintain your core starting in pregnancy, which helps to minimize or prevent many of the postpartum problems often thought of as being normal. You will also know how to properly heal your body after birth.

ABDOMINAL CHANGES DURING PREGNANCY

The changes the abdominal wall goes through in pregnancy and birth leave far more than cosmetic issues for women to deal with. Women should learn about these changes and how to manage them. By doing so, they will have the opportunity to make the best choices for their body in their pregnancy fitness and in their postpartum recovery.

There are three groups of abdominal muscles—the transversus abdominis muscles make up the deepest layer, then the oblique muscles (internal and external), and finally the rectus abdominis muscles, which are the outermost abdominals (see figure 4.1). They all attach via an aponeurosis, a broad sheet of dense connective tissue, to the linea alba, which is the connective tissue that holds the two rectus muscles in place. All the abdominal muscles face increasing stretch and strain in both pregnancy and birth, but it is the rectus abdominis muscles moving away from the midline as the belly grows that many consider to be the most visible and lasting change.

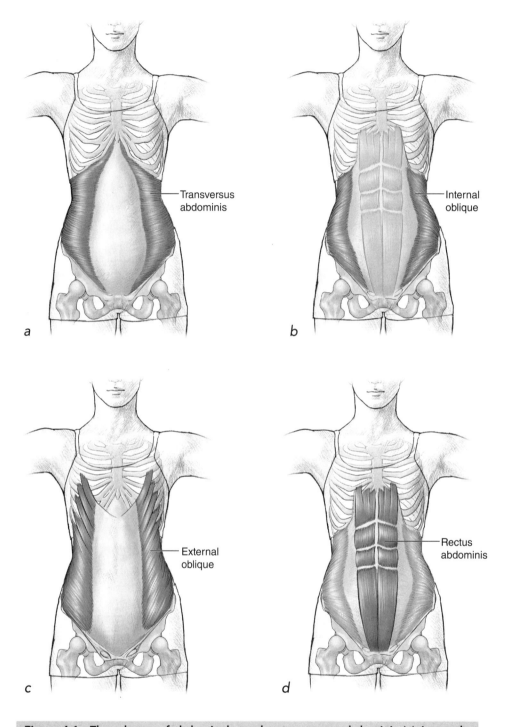

Figure 4.1   Three layers of abdominal muscles: transverse abdominis (a), internal and external obliques (b and c), and rectus abdominis (d).

In pregnancy, as the baby and belly grow, there is increased pressure on the linea alba. Over time, the linea alba thins and stretches (a normal response in pregnancy), allowing the two rectus muscles to move away from the midline. Before pregnancy, the muscles are never fused together, but rather they are supported in their position by the linea alba with a certain distance between the two straps of muscle. There has never been a true consensus on what is considered a normal inter-recti distance, but we know that the distance increases in pregnancy as a natural response to the growth of the baby and uterus. In approximately half of women, the rectus muscles return to their position once the baby is born, but about 40 percent of women have diastasis recti at six months postpartum (da Mota, Pascoal, Carita, and Bø 2014).

Diastasis recti (see chapter 1) is often considered to be an abnormal distance between the two rectus muscles and is most commonly characterized in pregnancy by the abnormal abdominal coning or doming you see when trying to sit up or roll down (see figure 4.2). While the postpartum poochy tummy is what many women dislike the most, it is the loss of function that trumps the inter-recti distance. The inability to create tension across the abdominal wall is where diastasis poses the real threat both during pregnancy and postpartum. When muscles themselves stretch beyond their optimal length and when the connective tissue thins, the abdominal wall can lose its ability to create the tension needed for core stability. Function is compromised and the ensuing compensations can create conditions such as back pain, pelvic girdle pain, and pelvic floor dysfunction.

The abdominal wall plays a role in managing pressures and forces in the body. Without the ability to generate and maintain tension using the abdominal wall, your ability to transmit force from your upper body to your lower body is compromised. Consequently, you may wind up using compensatory strategies such as changing your posture and overusing the obliques, hip flexors, and other muscle groups.

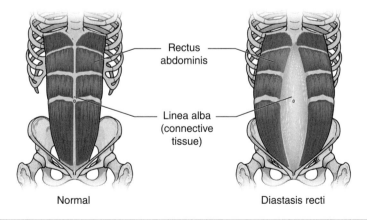

Rectus abdominis

Linea alba (connective tissue)

Normal

Diastasis recti

Figure 4.2 Diastasis recti.

As it stands now, women are uninformed about these abdominal challenges. No one is telling them what diastasis recti is, how to minimize it in pregnancy, or when and how to heal it. Women are finding out about it months or years later, often through social media, and then feel let down by their health care professionals and wonder why no one told them about it. Research is now pointing to the fact that every woman will have some degree of diastasis recti in or after pregnancy, but mainstream health care disregards it, viewing it only as a cosmetic issue. But it is more than that. Diastasis is non-optimal biomechanics. Because no information is shared with women in pregnancy and no one is checking for it postpartum, women are suffering and left to feel it is just a part of becoming a mother that they have to live with forever.

Fortunately, you have the opportunity in pregnancy to minimize the strain on the connective tissue, therefore minimizing the resulting diastasis recti and other dysfunctions. Paying attention to the way you stand, sit, and move will go a long way toward preserving your abdominal wall and overall core.

WHAT ARE THE CORE 4?

An understanding of the core and how it works is a great place to start when learning how you can minimize dysfunction in your core. We have introduced the Core 4 in previous chapters—they are the four muscles or muscle groups that form your deep core system and are together responsible for stabilization and control of movement. They are the transversus abdominis muscles, the multifidus muscles, the diaphragm, and the pelvic floor muscles (see figure 4.3). These muscles contract and co-contract in a certain pattern to ensure alignment, proper breathing, and coordination during a task. We'll return to the ABCs— alignment, breathing, and coordination— later in the chapter.

Transversus Abdominis

The transversus abdominis muscles form the deepest layer of the abdominal wall and connect in the front through an aponeurosis at the midline to the linea alba. This muscle plays a role in creating fascial tension between the segments of the spine and in the pelvis. It is anticipatory in nature (as are the diaphragm and pelvic floor), contracting milliseconds before the movement of your limbs or trunk. It co-contracts with the pelvic floor and last, but certainly not least, it is a forced expiratory muscle. This means it helps with blowing out during a cough or a sneeze.

The transversus abdominis muscle moves inward and outward (toward and away from the spine). As it does, it pulls the linea alba with it, creating tension along the midline. This tension is essential for helping return the postpartum abdominal wall to normal and is critical for healing a diastasis.

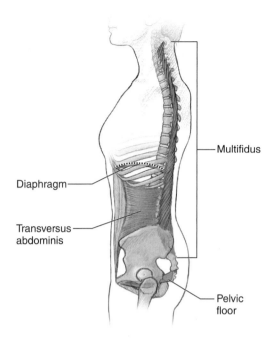

Multifidus

Diaphragm

Transversus abdominis

Pelvic floor

Figure 4.3　Core 4.

The ideal way to connect with the transversus abdominis is through the pelvic floor. We will show you how with the core breath a little later.

The transversus abdominis must exhibit varying amounts of tone throughout the day to help support the spine and internal organs during movement and at rest. Too much tone will create downward pressure on your pelvic organs, which can lead to incontinence, prolapse, or both. Too little tone or the inability to manage intra-abdominal pressure leads to a lack of support for the spine and abdomen. Pregnancy naturally stretches the transversus abdominis, affecting the muscle's ability to function. Paying attention to posture and alignment changes will better allow your transversus abdominis to maintain function throughout your pregnancy and afterward.

Posture and hormones are strong influences that affect the transversus abdominis. As the hormone relaxin is secreted, the linea alba becomes more lax to allow stretching to occur. Stretching of the structures of the abdominal wall is a natural response of the body to create space for the baby. The transversus abdominis itself becomes stretched, and moreover, because it inserts into the linea alba (which is itself becoming more lax), it loses a solid anchor to pull upon during muscle contraction, further challenging the support system.

Your growing uterus is putting quite a stretch on the entire abdominal wall and the transversus and rectus abdominis muscles have to give the most. The transversus abdominis is stretched beyond its optimal length, which makes it weaker and possibly ineffective in its roles as an expiratory muscle and in creating tension across the abdominal wall. Excessive stretch, like what happens during pregnancy, can interfere with the anticipatory action of the transversus abdominis, resulting in compensation from other muscles, especially the internal and external obliques, leading to their overuse. This can result in what is called *coning*, a doming or football-shaped bulge along the midline of your abdominal wall when you lean back or try to get up off the floor. This coning is indicative of diastasis recti, and is one reason why crunches are not recommended in pregnancy or as a postpartum recovery exercise. As you crunch up, there is an increase in intra-abdominal pressure that in pregnancy becomes increasingly difficult to manage.

While we are on the topic, one of the most common questions in prenatal and postpartum fitness is "Can I do crunches?" We first invite you to explore why you want to do crunches, or any exercise for that matter. What is your goal and how is this exercise bringing you closer to that goal? For many, it is believed that crunches are the way to flatten the midsection and is the best way to work the core. Crunches use only 20 percent of the rectus abdominis. With the changes to the alignment of the muscles, loss of tension in the linea alba, and compensatory strategies of the muscles in pregnancy, crunches become even less effective. Crunches round the shoulders (not what a pregnant or breastfeeding mom needs more of) and cause the rectus muscles to shorten and bulge outward. As this happens, the intra-abdominal pressure increases and can be damaging to the abdominal wall and pelvic floor. The next answer to the question "Can I do crunches?" is always, "I don't know...can you?" It's not about the exercise, but rather *how* you do the exercise that matters. Do the exercise and have a friend or trainer watch your abdomen. Also, pay attention to what you feel in your body when you do the exercise. If you can manage the pressures without doming or coning, you feel good doing the exercise, and it is bringing you closer to your goal, then great! Carry on.

Note, too, that getting up off the floor from a back-lying position is kind of like doing a crunch, and we want you to avoid that, too. So during pregnancy and in the early weeks postpartum, get up from and lower down to the floor by doing a "sexy slide." Instead of sitting and then leaning straight back to lower yourself onto the floor or crunching straight up to a sitting position to get up, sit on your left side first, then support yourself with your arms while you slide the left side of your body further down until your head touches the floor. Then roll over onto your back. To get up, roll to your side then use your arms to help press you up. Moving this way is great for your triceps and it will help protect your abdomen and pelvic floor from any unnecessary pressure on the connective tissue. Flexion will happen. You will be lying in bed and hear your baby cry and you will bolt out of bed, but don't panic! We aren't saying you can never flex or crunch again; we are simply suggesting you avoid it in pregnancy and while your Core 4 is healing. Then, gradually add flexion movements back in to your routine

BODY FACT

Intra-abdominal pressure is one of the natural forces within the body—we all have it and need it. In pregnancy, however, due to posture and alignment shifts, the influence of hormones, and all the other changes that occur, the core may lose some of its ability to manage increases in intra-abdominal pressure. This lack of proper function can result in back pain, pelvic girdle pain, and pelvic floor dysfunction. Following the guidelines on optimizing posture and alignment, moving with awareness, and retraining your core postpartum are great ways to help maintain your ability to manage intra-abdominal pressure.

if you choose to and can do it without doming or coning. Remember, it is not about the exercise, but rather how you do the exercise and how that exercise helps you achieve your goals.

Multifidus

The multifidus is a tiny little muscle that runs up each side of the spine from the sacrum. At every level, it attaches to the spinous processes of the vertebra, those little, protruding dinosaur-like bones that stick out when you bend your back. It is often overlooked, especially in fitness, but it is a critical muscle in the Core 4. It supports and protects the spine and pelvis and is engaged prior to movement in coordination with the pelvic floor muscles and the transversus abdominis. Weakness in the multifidus can be the cause of back pain, and back pain can cause this muscle to be weak—a frustrating pain–weakness cycle that is very common in pregnancy.

The multifidus is often shut down when there is lower-back pain and, because pregnant women experience more lower-back pain than non-pregnant women, we need to be aware of the impact of pregnancy on the multifidus. Also, the multifidus, like the other Core 4 muscles, is very sensitive to changes in your alignment and is often inhibited in pregnancy due to posture changes alone, with or without lower-back pain. This is another good reason to be mindful of your posture.

Diaphragm

The diaphragm is the major breathing muscle. Breathing is essential to life and good health, yet most people do it incorrectly. When you breathe, the diaphragm contracts and descends as you inhale. In response, the pelvic floor lengthens and descends and the transversus lengthens and expands outward. When you exhale, the movements are reversed. At least, that is what *should* happen. Unfortunately, our modern-day lifestyle is interfering with our ability to breathe properly, which then has a direct impact on our core function. We spend a large amount of time sitting in a slouched posture while we drive, while we work, and while we chill out in front of the TV. As a result, the diaphragm does not have the space to expand and descend. Furthermore, the pelvic floor does not have the opportunity to respond because it is shortened and tucked underneath the body while we sit.

Therefore, we tend to breathe up into our chest instead of into our side and back ribs. The pelvic floor and deep abdominals miss out on the beautiful movement with each breath and subsequently become compromised. When the rib cage is aligned optimally over the pelvis and when the sacrum and tailbone are out from the tucked position, the diaphragm and pelvic floor enjoy a synergistic ebb and flow throughout the day, which optimizes core function. When the rib cage is restricted and when the tailbone is tucked underneath us, breathing and overall function start to deteriorate.

In addition to the everyday poor posture described above, the posture changes in pregnancy have a direct influence on your diaphragm. As your belly grows and your center of gravity shifts, you will unknowingly try to counter this by leaning back, gripping your butt cheeks, and pressing your pelvis forward. This changes the alignment of the ribs in relation to the pelvis. Couple this with a baby that is taking up more and more space each day, and the diaphragm has a harder time descending on the inhale. This causes more of your breath to move into your upper chest as opposed to into your side ribs. When the diaphragm can't descend to its full capacity, the pelvic floor and transversus will start to lose out on the natural responsive movement they get with each breath as well.

Keep this in mind for your recovery as well. As a new mom you will spend a lot of time hunched over while carrying and nursing a baby. This posture can wreak havoc on the alignment and coordination between your diaphragm and pelvic floor. It is essential that you pay attention to your posture and your body alignment for optimal core function in pregnancy and postpartum.

Pelvic Floor

The pelvic floor, as you learned in chapter 3, is a collection of muscles, nerves, tendons, blood vessels, ligaments, and connective tissue all interwoven in the pelvis. It extends from the pubic joint in the front to the tailbone in the back and to the sitz bones (ischial tuberosities) on each side. It lengthens and lowers when you breathe in and rises and shortens as you breathe out in sync with the diaphragm.

The pelvic floor must have strength, endurance, timing, coordination, and control. It must work synergistically with the rest of the Core 4 to anticipate and prepare you for movement. It also must move synergistically to contribute to and help manage intra-abdominal pressure. Using the muscles of the pelvic floor with the diaphragm and transversus abdominis to modulate this pressure during exercise is critical for minimizing the effects of pregnancy and for your recovery after birth. It is also very important in helping to minimize diastasis, as too much intra-abdominal pressure is a contributor to the separation of the rectus muscles. Connecting with the pelvic floor is essential to generate tension through the abdominal wall. Learning how to do this in pregnancy will mean less discomfort as your body changes, a responsive pelvic floor for birth, and a quicker recovery postpartum.

The pelvic floor goes from supporting one to three pounds (0.5 to 1.5 kg) to nearly 10 times that amount in pregnancy. The changing angle of pull from posture changes causes the pelvic floor muscles to shorten, putting more of the weight directly on them instead of utilizing the pelvic bones for support. The tucked-under tailbone position common in pregnancy also inhibits the glutes. The pelvic floor and the glutes love working together, but their working relationship becomes challenged in pregnancy, leaving both in weakened states. In some women we will see the pelvic floor muscles become quite tight (hypertonic), in others we see them give up and become lax (hypotonic), and in a third group we see mixed tone where some muscles are really working hard while others have given up. And here again, with relaxin and other hormones coming into play on the sacroiliac joints, the pelvic floor faces significant challenges. These are some of the reasons we see an increase in incontinence, pelvic girdle pain, and lower-back pain in pregnancy.

Pregnancy brings many changes—hormone levels, a growing uterus, enlarged breasts, a stretched abdomen, extra weight on the pelvic floor, a shifting center of gravity, changes in collagen, ligament laxity, joint instability, and more! With all these changes, the Core 4 face many challenges as they try to maintain function. Muscles work best when they are at their optimum length. A muscle that is too short cannot generate as much power and the timing can be off. The same holds true for a muscle that is too long.

Pregnancy posture really is a key contributor to many of the common aches and pains of pregnancy and the resulting challenges such as diastasis recti, incontinence, pelvic organ prolapse, and pain. With the right preparation and awareness, you can minimize these changes, maintain core function in pregnancy, and return to a confident core postpartum!

PREPARE YOUR ABS FOR BIRTH

In order to prepare your body for birth, minimize the effects of the changes on your abdominal wall, and help ensure a better recovery postpartum, you can think about the ABCs—alignment, breathing, coordination—that we mentioned earlier. Proper alignment comes first, which will ensure optimal breathing patterns, which will then allow coordination among the Core 4 to do their many jobs, even when faced with the changes.

Alignment

The common posture seen in pregnancy is one where the tailbone starts to tuck under, the glutes become flat and inhibited, the shoulders round, the pelvis thrusts forward, and the rib cage sits behind the pelvis (see figure 1.1 in chapter 1). This results in nonoptimal alignment, puts an even greater strain on the abdominal wall, and makes you look more pregnant than you are. The good news is that with awareness and exercise, these shifts can be minimized or avoided all together. Stand sideways by a mirror with your feet pelvis-width apart. Back your pelvis up so it is over your heels and your weight is distributed through your heels with any overflow going into the midfoot rather than having the bulk of the weight in the forefoot. Now check that your ribs are over your pelvis and that your nipples are pointing forward and not up toward the sky. Last, make sure your ears are over your shoulders. See figure 1.1 in chapter 1 for an example of this proper alignment. It may feel like work to hold yourself there, and part of that is because your body has become accustomed to the lazier way of holding your body in space. The more you move, the less you sit, and with the right body awareness and exercise, this will become your new norm and will feel effortless while also allowing your Core 4 to work as they should.

Breathing

For something we do unconsciously throughout the day, it may seem odd to have to learn to breathe properly, but bad habits, pregnancy and birth, and insufficient daily movement cause the Core 4 to lose alignment, which interferes with optimal breathing. Once you have your posture and alignment in check, you can add in breath work to re-pattern effective breathing and maintain optimal Core 4 function.

The core breath exercise, which you will learn in chapter 6, is great to do daily on its own and also to integrate as part of your regular exercise routine. Proper breathing is key to minimizing the discomforts of pregnancy as well as ensuring a return to optimal core function postpartum. We know that women with incontinence and breathing problems have a higher risk of developing back pain and vice versa (Smith, Russell, and Hodges 2014). This is *huge*! Incontinence and diastasis rectus abdominis go hand in hand because they have similar causes, so proper breathing addresses at least two common problems.

Coordination

In fitness, there is a general rule of thumb to exhale on exertion. Now that you know about alignment and you know how to activate your core during an exhale, it is time to ensure you can coordinate that with movement and apply it to your exercises. Take the biceps curl for instance. Inhale and expand to prepare, then exhale to engage your core just before you curl the dumbbells up to your shoulders. This ensures the core is ready for the task at hand and trains the anticipatory element of the core. Finally, inhale and lower the dumbbells back down. It may seem easy, but coordinating the in and out breaths with pelvic floor activation and movement can be really challenging. Once you have it, you can turn almost any exercise into a powerful core exercise just by being purposeful with your breath.

A major contributor to diastasis rectus abdominis is birth itself. Birth is often portrayed with a woman on her back with her knees at her ears, and someone telling her to hold her breath and push using the Valsalva method (holding your breath while bearing down) or what is known as "purple pushing." Pushing the baby out while lying on your back is mechanically disadvantageous. Couple that with breath-holding and you have a pelvic floor and abdomen that literally can't handle the pressure. Instead, exhale through your pushes as much as possible with only a small breath hold at the end of the exhale if needed. It is also advised to push when *you* feel the urge as opposed to when someone tells you to push.

A modification to the core breath can be practiced in your last few weeks of pregnancy to reduce the challenge to your Core 4 during birth. Instead of picking up blueberries, as you learned in chapter 3, you will inhale to expand and then exhale through pursed lips while keeping that expansion and space in the pelvic floor. The pelvic floor needs to be able to stretch and lengthen in birth, so in this stage, thinking of picking up blueberries and contracting (shortening) the floor will be counterproductive.

The core breath is designed to help repattern and then maintain optimal breathing in pregnancy. It will also be the first exercise you do in your postpartum recovery, to repattern and retrain the Core 4, as you'll learn in chapter 6.

POSTPARTUM RECOVERY

Research has shown that any spontaneous healing of the abdominal wall occurs in the first eight weeks postpartum. Women are missing this optimal healing time because no one tells them about diastasis recti before or in pregnancy, and then they face a bigger challenge to healing. With the right awareness about alignment and exercise in pregnancy, recovery can begin before the baby is even born. All pregnant women will benefit from learning how to create a path for muscle memory postpartum.

Another healing strategy used in many cultures around the world which is increasing popularity in North America is abdominal wrapping. It is a gentle practice meant to support the pelvis and abdominal wall in the early weeks postpartum to aid in core restoration. The tissues in the abdominal wall and pelvic floor undergo tremendous stretch and strain in pregnancy and birth and need some support until their function is restored. Just as you would wrap injured tissue in an ankle sprain, you should wrap the injured tissues of the abdominal wall while you rebuild the Core 4. Wrapping the belly in the early weeks postpartum will provide physical support to the healing tissues and help encourage muscle realignment. This support, coupled with the core breath and restorative exercises to retrain the core, will help you efficiently restore your core. This is a simple concept that all women should know about, yet it is overlooked. As a result, many women unnecessarily deal with a lingering pooch, back pain, and pelvic floor dysfunction.

We recommend that you get an abdominal wrap during pregnancy so you can start wearing it right after birth and so you have it to wear during the

Take Action

During pregnancy, it's a good idea to check for diastasis recti. Following is a great self-test you can do while you're pregnant to help you get an idea of any loss of tensile ability in the abdominal wall. First, sit on the floor and place your hands behind you and slowly lower your upper body to the floor, using your hands to guide you. Look at your belly as you lower down and ask yourself these questions: Does it cone out like a football? Does it bulge just above your belly button? Does it stay flat and not change? Finally, repeat using the core breath—inhale to expand, then exhale to engage and lower yourself down. Did the doming disappear? If you see the doming or coning, it shows that the separation between the rectus muscles is happening. Remember, it is a normal response to pregnancy. If you can minimize or eliminate the doming or coning when you do the core breath, that's great! Keep doing that when you get out of bed, out of a comfy slouching position and anytime you are on your back and are unable to roll to the side.

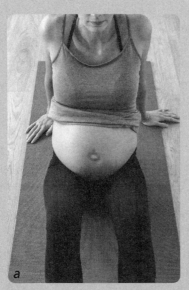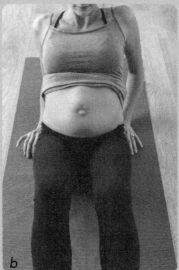

Checking for diastasis recti: (a) seated and (b) leaning back. Notice the coning after (b) leaning back.

most optimal healing time— the first eight weeks postpartum. Ideally, find one that is elastic so it can be placed around the pelvis and the abdomen. It is also important to find one that can adjust and shrink with you. Probably the most important aspect of postpartum belly wrapping is to put the wrap on from the bottom up. Many think of postpartum wrapping as "binding" or "waist training" and place the wrap around the waist only, which can create downward pressure on the pelvic floor. Ensure your wrap is placed around the hips first and then with an upward lift and with a gentle hug around the abdomen.

To find out if you have diastasis recti once you are no longer pregnant, perform the Postpartum Curl-Up Test (CUT). Be aware, however, that it is advised to wait until about 6 weeks postpartum to do this assessment. The steps are as follows:

1. Lie on your back with your knees bent and feet flat on the floor.
2. Press the index and middle fingers of one hand tightly together.
3. Keep your fingers straight with the fingertips pointing down.
4. Relax your abdominals.
5. Press the two joined fingers gently downward into the belly, with your fingers pointing toward the floor, just above the belly button.
6. Feel for the integrity of the connective tissue (linea alba). Does it feel mushy, stretchy, or tight? Can you push down until you feel your pulse?
7. Now feel for the separation: With your fingers still pressed together, tuck your chin and slowly lift your head off the floor as if starting a crunch. Feel for the edges of the recti coming together and "hug" your fingers. Measure at the first hint of hugging. Add more fingers and repeat if you do not feel the hug right away—this is an important step because most people take the first hug as their final measurement. Repeat from top to bottom of the midline from your sternum to your pubic bone.
8. Now feel for tension: Inhale to expand, exhale to engage. Is there a change in the tension of the linea alba under your fingertips?
9. Now feel for tension with the curl-up: Lie on your back with your knees bent and your feet flat on the floor. Slowly lift your head off the floor as if starting a crunch. Is there a bulge in your abdomen? Or does it feel mushy along the midline? Now lie back down, inhale to expand and prepare, then exhale to engage and slowly lift your head off the floor again. Did the tension along your abdomen stay when you lifted your head? Or did it bulge out or feel mushy again?

By definition, diastasis recti means separation of the rectus abdominis, but the condition involves much more than a gap between the two strap-like recti muscles. The inability to generate tension across the midline is the real challenge with this condition. As discussed earlier, the distance between the

BODY FACT

The linea alba, which directly translated means white line, is a fibrous structure that runs down the midline of the abdomen from the xyphoid process to the pubic symphysis. In pregnancy, this line turns brown in about 75 percent of women due to increased melanocyte-stimulating hormone made by the placenta. This hormone also causes melasma and darkened nipples in pregnancy. The brown color typically disappears within a few months after birth. The reason why some women get the line and others don't is unclear. Some believe it is more prevalent in women with darker skin or who are in the sun a lot. Regardless of if you get the line or not, it is not reflective of the sex of the baby, the health of the baby, or your health – it is simply something that happens—usually around the second trimester—to some and not to others.

recti muscles is informative, but as an outcome measure it really doesn't tell us much. There is a difference between a 3-finger and a 10-finger interecti distance, but most women are around 5 to 6 fingers postpartum. The real outcome measure is whether you can generate tension across that space between the 6-pack muscles. So if your midline feels mushy or soft, even when you exhale to engage, there is a lack of tension. If you saw a ridge or a cone-shaped bulge as you curled up, this also indicates a lack of tension.

In the curl-up test, if you are able to generate tension using one of the cues for your Core 4 and can hold the tension during the curl-up, you are considered to have a functional diastasis recti, which means your Core 4 will engage when you ask them to. A non-functional diastasis recti is when you cannot create tension, with or without cueing. Knowing if you are functional or non-functional becomes important when exercising, because you need to be able to generate tension in order to manage the loads of many exercises.

Seeing a pelvic floor physiotherapist during pregnancy and around six weeks after birth will help you better manage the changes of pregnancy, can help optimize your body for birth, and will help ensure the abdominal wall and pelvic floor are healing properly once your baby is born. A pelvic floor physiotherapist is a very valuable health guide that is not talked about; that needs to change. A pelvic floor physiotherapist should be a part of every pregnant woman's support team.

The abdomen gets all the glory in pregnancy and rightly so! We invite you to also let it shine in motherhood as well! It is unfortunately the part of the body women want most to change after having a baby. Perhaps with this information and the preventive and restorative recommendations we offer, women will take the awareness and make different choices – ones that minimize things like diastasis recti and also help heal it after baby is born.

II

Exercises to Prepare for and Recover From Birth

5

Stretch and Release Work

Pregnancy is an exciting time and presents some unique challenges to the mind, body, and spirit. The nine-month evolution is full of hormonal influences, physiological changes, and alterations to the body that may not always be welcome. A way to minimize the common discomforts that pregnancy can present is to incorporate daily stretch and release work. When preparing the body for birth, strength and endurance are important, but having supple, responsive muscles that allow space in the pelvis and that are able to yield, even while feeling discomfort, is essential! The pelvis, and its surrounding muscles, is definitely a key area of focus, but that doesn't mean the rest of the body is forgotten. Also note that performing your release work in a warm, quiet space will help optimize the process and allow your muscles the full opportunity to release and unwind. Release work for the entire body is essential—not just in pregnancy, but for life.

UPPER-BODY STRETCH AND RELEASE WORK

The key areas of the upper body you want to pay attention to are the neck and shoulders, the chest, and the obliques. The neck and shoulders take on a lot of strain with not only the alignment changes that are happening but also the increased sitting of our modern lifestyle. It is important to keep this area free of tension to avoid neck and shoulder pain, headaches, and stuck tissue. The chest is also faced with tension and strain due to the fact that most of the activities we do day to day involve working with things in front of us, so we are always reaching and leaning forward. The chest as a whole is tight, and when you add on to that the weight of the growing breasts, the alignment changes, and then all the breastfeeding and baby carrying that will happen, it can become a real source of held tension. The obliques are part of the abdominal wall, which we know faces significant change. Often, they are a muscle group that can start to be overworked when our overall core stability becomes challenged. The internal obliques rotate the trunk and bend it sideways, while the external obliques help pull the chest downward.

Tension + Integrity = Tensegrity

When looking at release work it is important to address the term *tensegrity*. This is a term that spawned from the work of architect Buckminster Fuller and it refers to forces of tension (provided by the muscles, tendons, ligaments, and fascia) that pull on the structure (the bones and joints) to help maintain stability and efficiency of movement.

Fascia is a web of connective tissue that runs seamlessly throughout the entire body. It wraps around every organ, muscle, bone, blood vessel, and nerve in the body and is literally what holds us together. Fascia facilitates or inhibits our ability to function and move as a body. It is located under the skin and is a three-dimensional web of support made up of collagen and elastin fibers that line up based on the lines of force in the body. Fascia is essentially adjustable tensegrity around all the bones in the body. Things like overuse, repetitive strain, and injury can all contribute to the fascia becoming disorganized, which can impair optimal movement. Because fascia is a seamless web running through the entire body, when fibers become "stuck" in one area of the body, movement can be impaired in another part of the body. Feeling tension in the shoulders might direct you to massage or bodywork that will target that area directly, but often the location of the tension is not where the problem is. Addressing the fascia system as a whole by incorporating whole-body movement and release work that considers the entire interconnected web will benefit your overall function and comfort in pregnancy, birth, and motherhood.

Ear to Shoulder Stretch

Focus and Benefits

As the breasts grow and the center of gravity shifts, you might feel more tension in the neck and shoulders. This stretch helps relieve that tension and is great for everyone, even those who are not pregnant.

Equipment

Stability ball or chair

Description

- Sit on a stability ball or chair with a neutral pelvis (or you can stand with a neutral pelvis) and allow your left ear to fall toward your left shoulder.
- Close your eyes and enjoy the lengthening you feel on the right side of your neck and shoulders. Hold for 10 to 30 seconds.
- For a deeper stretch, extend the opposite arm down the side of your body.
- To come out of the stretch, slowly drop your chin toward your chest and then bring the head back to center.
- Repeat on the other side and continue for three to five sets.

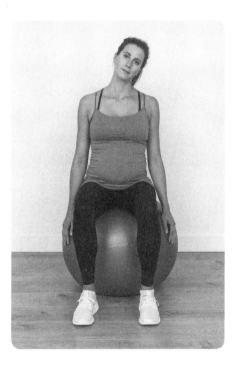

Rotate and Reach Stretch

Focus and Benefits

Motherhood requires an increase in many of our typical movements, including rotation. Rotation is a movement generated by the midback or thoracic area which can get very stiff with the posture changes we have discussed. It is also not a movement we do regularly. By adding in some rotation and reaching movements, you will be better prepared for the many times you will need those movements in motherhood. This stretch also helps create length and release in the torso for better breathing and freedom of movement in general.

Equipment

Stability ball or chair

Description

- Sit on a chair or stability ball with a neutral pelvis.
- Straighten your left arm and reach it gradually up to the ceiling as you rotate your torso to the left.
- Only go as far as you can without letting the right butt cheek come off the ball or chair.
- Hold for a count of 3-5 seconds then return to the starting position.
- Repeat on the other side.

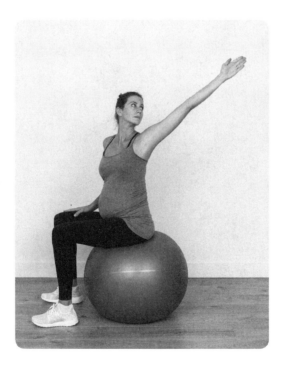

Shoulder and Chest Stretch With Strap

Focus and Benefits

The neck and shoulders are tight in most people, pregnant or not. We can all use some movement to open the chest and free up tension in the shoulders. This is a great dynamic stretch to do just that.

Equipment

Yoga strap

Description

- Stand with a neutral pelvis and grasp your strap in each hand slightly wider than shoulder width with palms facing down.
- Keeping the arms straight, lift the arms up and over the head until the band is no longer visible.
- Hold there for a few breaths and return to start.
- Repeat 10 times.

Safety Considerations

If you have any existing shoulder injuries or challenges, reduce the range of motion and don't hold the stretch. If your shoulder continues to bother you in this stretch, discontinue.

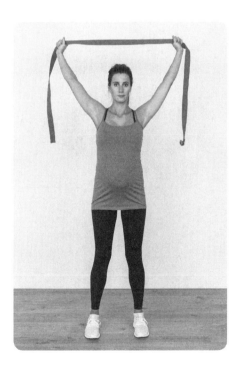

Standing C-Stretch

Focus and Benefits

The amount of sitting we do on a daily basis, coupled with the nonoptimal core-stability compensations we often see in pregnancy, can mean rigidity in the torso, especially in the obliques. This is a great way to create length in the side body and free up space for better breathing.

Equipment

Chair or wall (optional)

Description

- Stand next to the wall or chair (if using) with your right leg (the inside leg) about one foot away from the wall or chair (the image shows the stretch without the chair or wall).
- Place your right hand on the wall just below shoulder height or on the top of the chair (if using). Alternatively, link hands as shown in the photo.
- Cross your left foot over your right foot and allow the left hip to move away from the wall as you reach your left arm up and over your head.
- Your body will curve away from the wall in a C shape. Imagine your left side as an expanding slinky. Hold for 10 to 30 seconds.
- Repeat on the other side and continue for three to five sets.

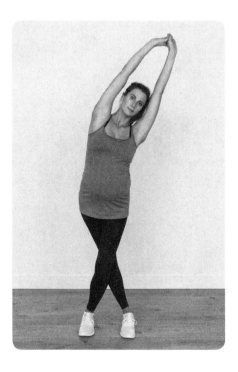

Seated Chest Stretch Over Stability Ball

Focus and Benefits

Many people would benefit by opening up the chest, especially pregnant women. This stretch is also great after nursing your little one. The roundness of the ball helps increase the stretch while allowing it to be restful.

Equipment

Stability ball

Description

- Nudge your ball into a corner or against a wall.
- Sit on the floor in front of the ball in a semireclined position with your feet on the floor in front of you.
- Clasp your hands behind your neck.
- Rest your head on the ball and allow your elbows to open to the sides and your chest to expand. Hold for 10 to 30 seconds.
- Do three to five sets.

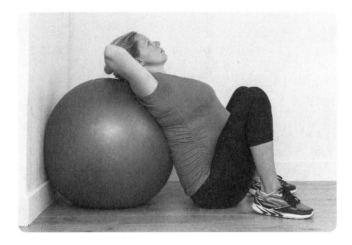

Side-Lying Stretch Over Ball

Focus and Benefits

This is one stretch that you will truly love to do. It is relaxing and lengthening and a great stress reliever.

Equipment

Small, semi-inflated ball or a small cushion and mat

Description

- Assume a side-seated position on the floor. Begin on your right side.
- Take the ball and place it between the top of your pelvis and the bottom your rib cage (on your waist) on your right side.
- Slowly lie down on your right side with the ball between you and the floor.
- Rest your head on the right arm and bend the right leg (the bottom leg) for support.
- Lengthen the left leg (the top leg) straight out and reach the left arm (the top arm) over your head.
- Hold for 30 to 90 seconds and repeat on the other side.

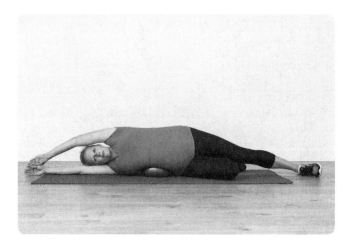

LOWER-BODY STRETCH AND RELEASE WORK

When stretching and releasing the lower body, the hamstrings, inner thighs, psoas, calves, and feet are all important. Sitting shortens the hamstrings, which can then lead to pulling the pelvis into that nonoptimal posterior pelvic tilt. The inner thighs are a place where many hold a lot of tension, and releasing them can help release the pelvic floor as well. The psoas muscles (you have two of them, one on either side) run from the base of the thoracic spine over the top of the pelvis to the top of the femur. They are the only muscles that join the top and bottom halves of the body. Tight psoas muscles can wreak havoc on the position of the pelvis and the rib cage, restrict space in the pelvis, and even interfere with labor. Becoming aware of your psoas muscles and nurturing them with release work daily in pregnancy will ensure your pelvis has space and freedom to support your baby in pregnancy and allow labor to unfold in the most optimal way.

Heeled shoes, restrictive footwear, and long periods of sitting can cause pain and discomfort in the feet and tightness in the calves, which can cause alterations in gait leading to compensations in the pelvis. Releasing tension in the lower legs and feet is a great way to maintain mobility in the lower body. Here are some key ways to facilitate freedom of movement in the lower body throughout pregnancy.

Feet on Ball Stretch

Focus and Benefits

Rolling your feet over a ball is such an amazing way to relieve tension and release "stuck" tissue in the feet, which can interfere with gait.

Equipment

Massage ball or tennis ball

Description

- Roll, rock, and press the foot on the ball for up to one minute.
- Repeat on other side.
- Do multiple times a day.

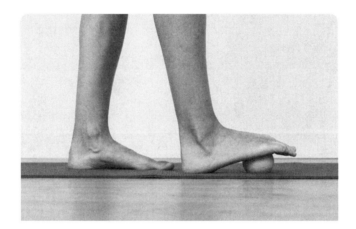

Calf Stretch

Focus and Benefits

The more length you have in your calves, the longer your foot can stay on the ground as you walk. This flexibility translates to greater efficiency and better pushoff. It also means more length in the back of the legs so the pelvis can find and stay in a neutral position with ease.

Equipment

Rolled towel or yoga mat, or foam roller cut in half lengthwise.

Description

- Place your rolled towel, mat, or foam roller on the floor.
- Place the ball of your right foot on the left end of the towel, mat, or roller. The right heel remains on the floor and the leg is straight.
- Step forward with the left leg until you feel a good stretch in the right calf and hold for 10 to 30 seconds.
- Repeat on the other side and continue for three to five sets.
- Try this without shoes for an even better stretch.

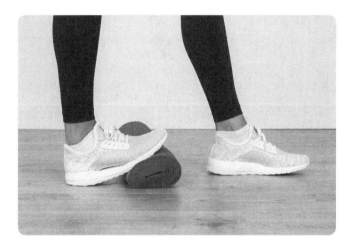

Adductor Stretch on Stability Ball

Focus and Benefits

Length in the inner thighs can help keep the pelvis free to move as it needs to in labor. This stretch is also one you can do in early labor to help encourage your baby to move into the pelvis.

Equipment

Stability ball or chair

Description

- Sit on a stability ball or chair with a neutral pelvis. Roll slightly forward on the ball or sit at the front edge of the chair.
- Extend the left leg straight out to the side.
- Reach the left leg away as you roll slightly to the right on the ball or chair and hold for 10 to 30 seconds.
- Repeat on the other side and continue for three to five sets.

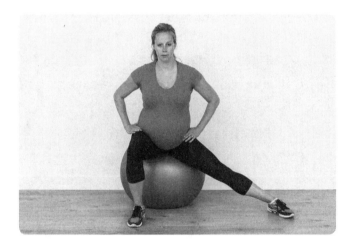

Hip Flexor Stretch on Stability Ball

Focus and Benefits

As we mentioned in the last stretch, opening and releasing the front of the pelvis will help optimize the position of the pelvis and facilitate your baby moving into and out of the pelvis on birth day.

Equipment

Stability ball or chair

Description

- Place your right butt cheek on the ball or chair with your right leg in front and your left leg stretched behind you, similar to a lunge position.
- Hold 10 to 30 seconds.
- Repeat on other side and continue for three to five sets

Safety Considerations

Wedge the ball against a wall if you need more stability.

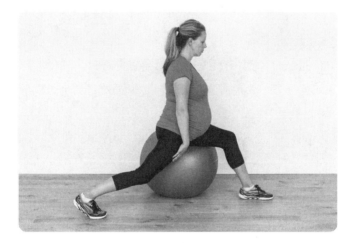

Focus and Benefits

This stretch targets the piriformis, the muscle that attaches from the sacrum (the triangular bone in your pelvis) to the femur (the thigh bone). Because it passes just behind the pelvic floor, tightness in the piriformis can influence the pelvic floor muscles and the bones of the pelvis. Releasing the piriformis will allow the sacrum to be in its optimal position, which will support proper pelvic floor function as well.

Equipment

Chair with hard surface

Description

- Sit on the chair with a neutral pelvis.
- Place your left ankle on your right knee, keeping the left foot flexed.
- Keeping a neutral pelvis and the sternum lifted, hinge forward at the hips until you feel a stretch deep in your hip and buttocks.
- Hold 10 to 30 seconds.
- Repeat on other side and continue for three to five sets.

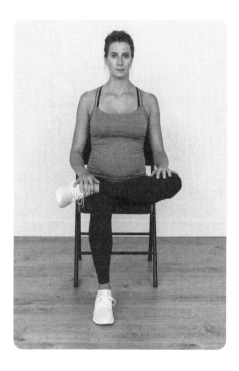

Hamstring Stretch With Strap

Focus and Benefits

The hamstrings originate from the sitz bones, formally called the ischial tuberosities. These are the bones you feel in your butt cheeks. When the hamstrings are tight they can pull on the sitz bones and encourage the pelvis to tip backwards (not ideal alignment of the pelvis). This stretch is designed to bring length to the hamstrings while the pelvis is in a neutral position.

Equipment

Yoga block or pillow, mat, and a yoga strap

Description

- Lie down on your mat with your head on a yoga block or a pillow.
- Find your neutral pelvis. This is where the hip bones and the pubic joint are in the same frontal plane.
- Hook a strap around the ball of your right foot and hold the strap in each hand.
- Keep the right leg straight while lifting it up toward the ceiling until you feel the pelvis start to tip back. This is a sign that your pelvis is moving out of a neutral position, so stop there. Keep the back of the left leg on the mat.
- Think of "nodding" the pubic joint toward the floor and of reaching the right sitz bone toward the bottom edge of the mat.
- Hold for 10 to 30 seconds.
- Repeat on other side and continue for three to five sets.

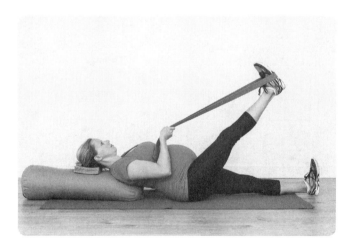

Psoas Release With Bolster

Focus and Benefits

The psoas muscle, when tight or when holding on to fear, can pull the spine forward, which in turn thrusts the rib cage forward (out of ideal alignment). It can also pull the femur bone (thigh bone) forward, which causes the pelvis to tip backwards (out of ideal alignment). Releasing the psoas can help encourage optimal alignment and create space in the pelvis for your baby to settle into and eventually move out of.

Equipment

Yoga bolster or stack of pillows, mat, and a towel or block

Description

- From a side-seated position, lie onto the bolster so that the bottom edge of the bolster is just above the bottom edge of your bra.
- Roll over onto your back so the bottom edge of the bolster is above the top of your bra strap and between the shoulder blades.
- Rest your head on another towel or block if needed, and rest your arms at your sides.
- Close your eyes and just relax and soften.
- This is not a "doing exercise" but an "allowing exercise." As you rest in this position you are working to allow your ribs to lower toward the floor so that they are neutral relative to the pelvis. Ideally, the bottom of the rib cage and the top of the pelvis will be in the same frontal plane.
- Try to relax in this position for five minutes.

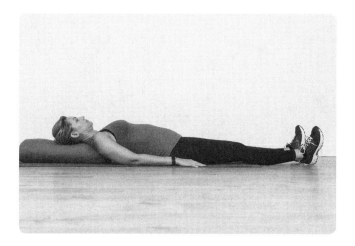

PELVIC FLOOR

Probably one of the most important parts of the body to stretch and release in preparation for birth is the pelvic floor. This is an area of the body that undergoes significant change in pregnancy and birth, yet it gets little attention. If anything is shared with women about the pelvic floor it is limited to "do your Kegels." While this is better than nothing, it certainly does not address the needs of the pelvic floor during pregnancy and birth or as a busy mom. Kegels can play a role in pelvic-floor wellness, but they are not for everyone. Many people actually need to focus on the relaxation portion or the letting go portion of a Kegel as opposed to the contraction portion.

Down training is a term often applied to learning how to relax the pelvic floor, which can be accomplished through visualization, stretching the surrounding muscles, myofascial release work, and perineal massage.

Posterior Pelvic Floor Release

Focus and Benefits

A common holding pattern that develops in pregnancy is a gripping or tensing of the posterior muscles of the pelvic floor, which can encourage a posterior tilt to the pelvis. This tension can also result when the pelvis is held in a posterior tilt (think of sitting slouched for the majority of the day). When we release these muscles, the pelvis has more freedom to find and stay in neutral alignment.

Equipment

Chair with a hard surface and a tennis or massage ball

Description

- Sit on a hard chair with a neutral pelvis.
- Lift your left butt cheek up and find your sitz bone.
- Place the ball in between your right sitz bone and your anus.
- Lower the butt cheek back down with the ball in place and hold 30 to 60 seconds.
- Repeat on other side.
- We have shown the ball to help you see where it goes but ideally, it will not be visible during the exercise.

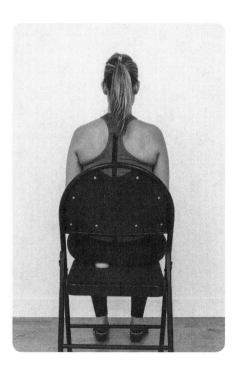

Perineum Release

Focus and Benefits

The perineum is the area between the vagina and the anus and is prone to tearing in childbirth. Becoming familiar with sensations of discomfort in the perineum and learning to yield to the discomfort and relax the area are important during birth. Become aware of your perineum in pregnancy and learn to release the tension there as you prepare for birth.

Equipment

Chair with a hard surface and a pool noodle

Description

- Sit on the chair with a neutral pelvis.
- Place a pool noodle lengthwise along the perineum.
- Hold for 30 to 60 seconds and breathe deeply. Work at softening and letting go of tension in the pelvic floor, the glutes, and the inner thighs.

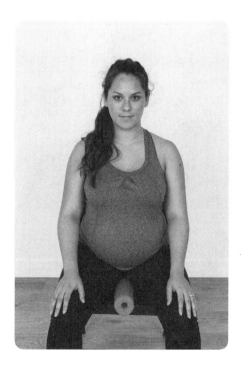

Perineal Massage

Focus and Benefits

Perineal massage is a practice that most women do to help avoid tearing. While studies have shown that perineal massage can play a role in reducing the likelihood of tearing, the practice is also about helping you teach your pelvic floor to respond appropriately to sensations of stretch, pressure, and discomfort. This is done in the last three to five weeks of pregnancy only.

Equipment

Rolled towels

Description

- Sit in a semi-reclined position on your bed with small, rolled-up towels under each butt cheek. This gives space for the sacrum to be free. (Take this towel trick with you into birth as well. If you choose or find yourself in the lithotomy position, have your partner or doula place the small rolled up towels under your butt cheeks so your sacrum can be free to move as needed).
- Lubricate your thumbs and your vulva.
- Insert your thumbs into your vagina.
- Press your thumbs out and up in a U shape and then hold at the top of the U.
- Hold for 5 to 10 seconds.
- You should feel a stretch, some pressure, and slight discomfort, but no pain.
- Breathe deeply and learn to soften and release tension as you feel the discomfort.
- Repeat for up to 10 minutes.

In fitness activities, it is natural to want to know how to increase the difficulty in order to progress. We challenge you to think differently when it comes to stretch and release work. Instead of thinking how to increase the intensity, simply allow yourself more time in a pose or a release exercise. Extending the time in a pose is actually a progression, but your mindset should be focused on the purpose—releasing tension— rather than increasing the difficulty or feeling a stretch more intensely.

In this busy world we live in, it can be hard to slow down. Taking the time to release tension in the body is a treat that many do not enjoy. In pregnancy it is not only a treat but also an essential tool that will help you in labor and birth. Learning to yield and soften and release against discomfort is critical because it is what you need to do in labor and birth. Challenge yourself to take the time.

For those who need to see progress and understand that what they are doing is making improvements, you can use your "edge" as a guide. When performing the stretch and release work, find your edge (the point of discomfort) and stay there. If you feel your edge subside during the exercise, that's good—that means you are releasing tension! You can then find a new edge by moving deeper into the stretch and eventually go on to create space and release tension in the new position.

6

Strengthening the Core

Our modern-day lifestyle is increasingly sedentary, which means many women are going into pregnancy and birth with nonoptimal core function. As we have discussed in previous chapters, the amount of sitting we do means the core muscles become weaker, and when that weak core is loaded to extremes at the gym, something's gotta give. Many times, it is the lower back or the pelvis that sends out distress signals such as pain or a leaky bladder. Pregnancy and birth add another element of intense demand to the core, leading to back pain, pelvic floor challenges, difficulty in labor, and abs that remain stretched and weak postpartum. Your core needs to work very hard throughout your pregnancy, so challenging it appropriately will ensure it is ready to do its jobs on birth day and in motherhood!

Your core is made up of an inner unit, called the Core 4 (see chapter 2), as well as other muscles surrounding the pelvis. All your core muscles are undergoing constant change as your baby grows and are being stretched beyond optimal length. The most visible changes in pregnancy and after are seen in the abdomen. While the belly is often shown off with pride as the baby grows in pregnancy, it often becomes the part of the body most women want to change or hide postpartum. The fitness industry has perhaps led pregnant women and new moms astray by ignoring appropriate movement and exercise that both prepares and restores the core and by focusing on getting the pre-baby body back after birth.

It is no secret that a fit, functional, and well-trained body will perform better during physically demanding events. Birth is a very physical event and you must train your core properly. By using the core breath and exercises provided in this chapter, you will have the core strength and the endurance to manage labor well. A conditioned core means abdominals that can assist the uterus in pushing the baby out. It means a pelvic floor that can be responsive to the changing needs of labor and have both strength and the ability to yield. A conditioned core means a strong and supple psoas muscle that has length and softness to allow space in the pelvis with no tension or fear getting in the way. A conditioned core also means a strong and confident body that can adapt and allow birth to happen. You are preparing for an amazing event and the exercises in this chapter will help you build strength, endurance, and suppleness in your core. Use them to prepare, recover, and restore.

The goal of core training in pregnancy is not to build a 6-pack but to work the core unit in a functional way that develops strength and endurance without rigidity and in ways that help minimize diastasis recti and maintain optimal function of the pelvic floor. Many people, especially women, believe that engaging the core or holding the abdominal muscles tight all day helps build strength. On the contrary, this practice creates constant pressure downward on the pelvic floor and can create tension or holding patterns in the core that can actually interfere with birth. For best results, instead of holding in your abs all day, you should be working on activating your core in coordination with your breathing during movement and developing an awareness of letting go of tension when you are resting.

We have compiled a collection of really great core exercises for you to use throughout your pregnancy. The first eight exercises will not only be done in pregnancy but are also your best recovery exercises! They are to be done progressively over the first eight weeks postpartum to retrain your Core 4. The beauty of these particular exercises is that by doing them in pregnancy you will already know how to do them, so when it comes time to use them for your recovery, you just go back to the first exercise—the core breath—and then gradually progress week by week without having to learn a whole new set of exercises.

New moms want to lose weight and flatten their tummy as soon as possible after the baby arrives, but we urge you to respect the need to heal, rest, and retrain the core before moving on to exercises like boot camp or running. These are activities you can go back to in time, but choosing them as your first activities and overlooking the core retraining will unfortunately move you further from your goal of a functional core. With an understanding of the core and how to use it best in pregnancy, your body can adapt more appropriately to the changes in pregnancy, facilitate labor, and look and feel amazing postpartum.

Let's take a look at the exercises you can use to get your core ready for labor and motherhood.

Core Breath

Focus and Benefits

The core breath is the ultimate foundational exercise. It trains the Core 4 to work as they should with synergy between the diaphragm, pelvic floor, deep abdominals, and multifidus. The core breath is done not only on its own but also while performing other exercises to really bring awareness of the inner core unit into movement. You will do the core breath regularly throughout pregnancy; it is also the very first restorative exercise you will do postpartum.

Equipment

Stability ball

Description

- Sit on a stability ball with a neutral pelvis (this can also be done lying on your side or on your back).
- Put one hand on the side of your ribs and the other hand on your belly.
- Breathe into your hands. Inhale to expand—feel the rib cage expand, feel the pelvic floor expand (you may feel fullness in your perineum), and feel the abdomen expand outward.
- Exhale through pursed lips and voluntarily contract your pelvic floor using imagery to engage. For example, imagine picking up a blueberry with your vagina and anus or imagine sucking a milkshake through a straw with your vagina, or imagine lifting your perineum up toward the crown of your head.

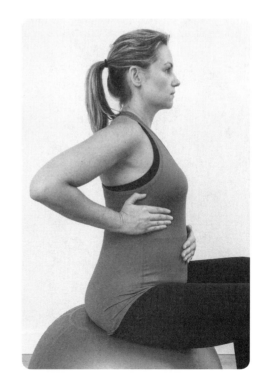

- Inhale to expand again and let the pelvic floor contraction subside (imagine letting go of the blueberry).
- Repeat for 10 to 30 breath cycles.
- Apply the Inhale to Expand, Exhale to Engage practice, as we learned in chapter 4, to any movement to ensure your core is active and ready. Experiment with different cues, and remember to use a cue every time you exhale to engage. It turns almost any exercise into a core exercise!

Do the core breath three times per day for one to two minutes each time to maintain optimal core function and to really get the coordination of this ex-

(continued)

ercise imprinted in your mind. Try it with different cues and then continue with the one that is best for you. Remember the modification in the weeks before birth. Inhale to expand then exhale and keep the expansion to mimic what you will do in labor. After your baby is born, restart the regular core breath within the first few days postpartum to help increase circulation and regenerate tone, strength, and function to the Core 4. We have said it many times…you need to re-train before you train and the core breath exercise is your biggest ally! It stimulates circulation and nerve growth factor to help optimize healing in the pelvic floor. It can help recover any loss of sensation that may have resulted from labor and it helps get as much oxygen as possible into the body to help heal the tissues. The best news is that you can, and should, use this powerful exercise for life!

Increase Difficulty

Try this exercise in a standing position.

Take Action

Your body instinctively knows how to push, and the urges you will feel are similar to those you feel when having a bowel movement. Think about it for a moment: no one taught you how to defecate, your body just responded to the urges. It is the same with birth, but often fear, which causes our tight muscles, gets in the way.

Find an environment where you feel safe and will not face a lot of interruptions so you can relax. Use the core breath inhale to relax your pelvic floor and create space. On the exhale, instead of doing a Kegel or picking up blueberries, you will keep the space you just created and send your breath down to your vagina while you let a little breath exhale from pursed lips. You will feel fullness in your perineum as you practice. Think of it as a modified core breath used to prepare to push. You can also visualize your baby coming down as you send your breath to guide him or her.

You can safely practice this push prep technique every time you have a bowel movement, and when you get to 36 weeks, you can start practicing in other labor positions like side-lying and on all fours (quadruped).

Bridge

Focus and Benefits

The bridge is one of the great glute exercises. Doing it daily in your pregnancy will help you build strong glutes, which helps with optimal pelvic alignment and optimizing the pelvic floor. Postpartum, bridges are fantastic because they offer a gentle inversion and encourage circulation to the healing pelvic floor.

Equipment

Mat and a small ball, such as a bender ball, or a small cushion or towel

Description

- Lie on your back with your knees bent, feet pelvis-width apart, and shins vertical (a).
- Find a neutral pelvis position where the pubic joint and the hip bones are in the same plane and you have a small curve in your lower back.
- Place a small ball, cushion, or towel between your thighs.
- Inhale to expand and prepare.
- Exhale to engage then press your hips up toward the ceiling (b).
- Inhale to expand as you lower your hips back down.

Safety Considerations

From the second trimester onward, place a wedge or pillows under your head and shoulders to keep your head above your heart.

Increase Difficulty

- In pregnancy, place a small sandbag weighing up to five pounds (2 kg) on your pelvis for more weight.
- In pregnancy, you can extend one leg.
- In pregnancy, you can try this with a BOSU ball (with the dome up) under your feet.
- When doing this exercise in the first eight weeks postpartum, simply do the base exercise and do not do anything to increase the difficulty.

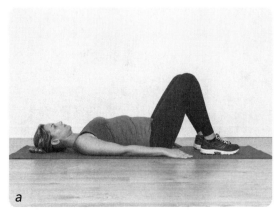

a

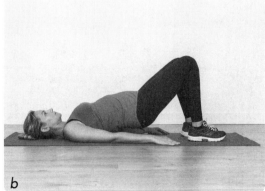

b

Clam Shell

Focus and Benefits
- Builds strength and endurance in the glutes and lateral hip muscles
- Trains your body for a side-lying birth position
- Prepares you for recovery. Note that this is also a key restorative exercise, and learning it in pregnancy means you don't have to learn a new exercise postpartum.

Equipment
Mat

Description
- Lie on your side with your knees bent a little less than 90 degrees. Ensure your hips and ankles are stacked— top hip directly over bottom hip and top ankle resting on bottom ankle *(a)*.
- Inhale using core breath to expand and prepare.
- Keeping your ankles pressed together, exhale to engage and then lift the top knee away from the bottom knee. This is a small movement of the hip with no movement anywhere else—only the knee lifts with the rotation occurring at the hip joint. Keep the pelvis still and controlled *(b)*.
- Inhale and lower the knee back down with control.

Increase Difficulty
- In pregnancy, use a resistance band around your thighs for greater resistance.
- In pregnancy, increase the length of time you hold your knee up to help build greater endurance.
- When doing this exercise in the first eight weeks postpartum, simply do the base exercise and do not do anything to increase the difficulty.

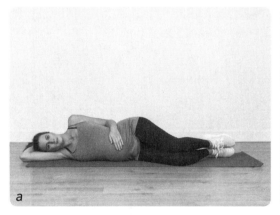
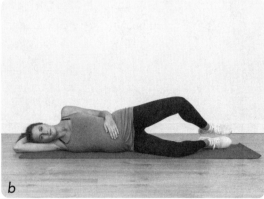

a

b

Side-Lying Bent-Knee Lift

Focus and Benefits

- Builds strength and endurance in the glutes and lateral hip muscles
- Prepares you for a side-lying birth position
- Prepares you for recovery. Note that this is also a key restorative exercise, and learning it in pregnancy means you don't have to learn a new exercise postpartum.

Equipment

Mat

Description

- Lie on your side with your knees and hips bent at 90 degrees or at slightly less than 90 degrees (as shown) and ensure your hips and ankles are stacked—top hip directly over bottom hip and top ankle resting on bottom ankle *(a)*.
- Inhale to expand and prepare.
- Exhale to engage and then lift the top leg toward the ceiling away from the bottom leg *(b)*.
- Inhale and lower the leg back down with control.

Increase Difficulty

- In pregnancy, use a resistance band around your thighs for resistance.
- In pregnancy, increase the length of time you hold your leg up to help build greater endurance.
- When doing this exercise in the first eight weeks postpartum, simply do the base exercise and do not do anything to increase the difficulty.

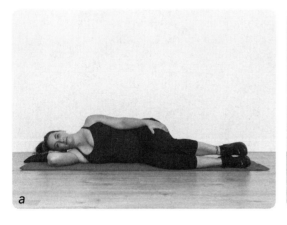
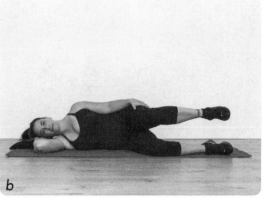

a

b

Squat

Focus and Benefits

- Builds strength and endurance in the quads, hamstrings, and glutes
- Trains your body using a functional movement
- Prepares you for squatting during labor

Equipment

Stability ball if desired

Description

- Stand with your feet pelvis-width apart and pointing straight ahead *(a)*.
- Inhale to expand as you hinge at the hips, send your bum back, and bend at the knees. Keep your weight in your heels *(b)*.
- Exhale to engage as you straighten your legs to press back up.
- Work in the 12 to 15 rep range and aim to complete one to two sets (see the workouts for more detail on sets and reps).
- You may also work at holding a static squat position, where you lower down and then hold the squat for 10 to 30 seconds.

Safety Considerations

As you learn the squat you may wish to do it with a stability ball behind you.

Increase Difficulty

- In pregnancy, try squatting on a BOSU with the dome up for a greater challenge. You may want to take a wider stance where the feet are placed more toward the sides of the BOSU. Ensure that your knees do not track forward over your toes. Note that this is not to be done in the second or third trimester; the added instability can increase the risk of falling.
- When doing this exercise in the first eight weeks postpartum, simply do the base exercise and do not do anything to increase the difficulty.

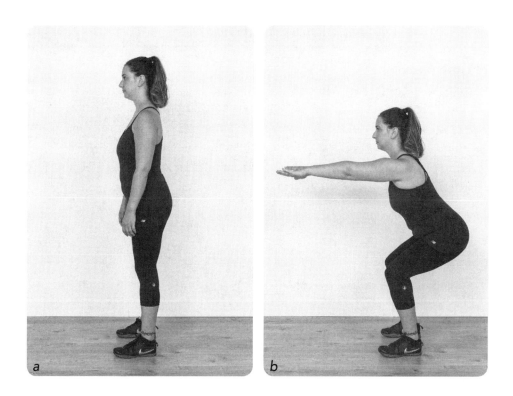

a

b

CHALLENGE YOURSELF Place a BOSU dome-up on the floor. Sit on the dome so that your perineum is at the center of the top of the BOSU. Place your feet pelvis-width apart on the floor and pointing straight forward, and with your shins vertical. Inhale to prepare. Then exhale to engage and stand up, ensuring you keep your weight in your heels and your shins as vertical as possible. You can practice this movement throughout the day as well. Every time you stand up from a seated position be purposeful, try to keep your shins vertical, and push up with your weight in your heels to really fire up the glutes and enjoy the booty benefits!

Seated March on Stability Ball

Focus and Benefits

- Trains the Core 4 to work as they should with synergy between the diaphragm, pelvic floor, deep abdominals, and multifidus
- The stability ball adds an element of instability to challenge balance and build the muscles that support the pelvis
- In the fifth week postpartum, starts retraining the core in an upright position and works on pelvic stability

Equipment

Stability ball

Description

- Wedge a stability ball into a corner and sit on the ball with a neutral pelvis. Place your feet pelvis-width apart on the floor and your hands gently resting on the sides of the ball.
- Inhale to expand and prepare.
- Exhale to engage and lift one foot about one or two inches off the floor. Keep the pelvis neutral; do not tuck it under and flatten your lower back.
- Inhale to expand and lower the foot back down.
- Repeat on other side.

Safety Considerations

Keep hands on sides of ball for stability.

Increase Difficulty

- Take the ball out of the corner and lean against the wall or away from the wall completely to increase instability.
- Take your hands off of the ball.
- Add in some alternate arm movements as you lift your leg.
- When doing this exercise in the first eight weeks postpartum, simply do the base exercise and do not do anything to increase the difficulty.

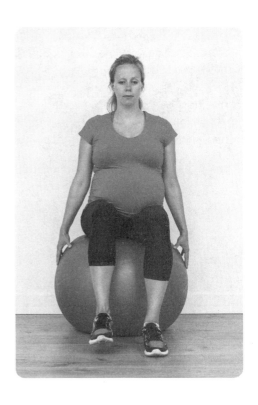

Standing One-Leg Transfer

Focus and Benefits

- Trains the Core 4 to work as they should with synergy between the diaphragm, pelvic floor, deep abdominals, and multifidus
- Prepares you for a staggered-stance standing position in labor
- Builds strength in the lateral hip muscles
- Restores stability in the pelvis when used postpartum
- Prepares you for return to running postpartum

Description

- Stand with your feet pelvis-width apart and with a neutral pelvis. Your hands can be on your hips or hanging at your sides (a).
- Inhale to expand and prepare.
- Exhale to engage and bend your knee while you lift your right foot four to six inches off the floor without allowing the pelvis to tilt or tuck under (b).
- Inhale to expand and lower the foot back down.
- Repeat on other side.

Safety Considerations

Place one hand on a wall if you feel you need more stability.

Increase Difficulty

- Keep your leg lifted for five to ten seconds.
- At the same time as you lift your foot off the floor, lift the opposite arm up.
- When doing this exercise in the first eight weeks postpartum, simply do the base exercise and do not do anything to increase the difficulty.

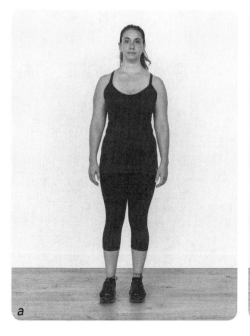
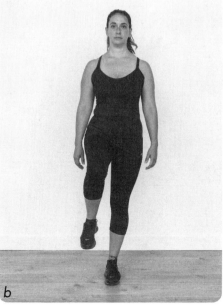

a

b

Lunge

Focus and Benefits

- Builds strength and muscular endurance in quads, hamstrings, and glutes
- Trains the body for a functional movement
- Prepares you for asymmetric standing birth positions

Equipment

Stability ball if desired

Description

- Stand with your right foot forward and your left foot behind you with the toes of your left foot on the floor and the heel up so you are in a split stance. If using a stability ball, place it between your low back and a wall behind you (a).
- Inhale to expand as you bend your right leg to lower down, pressing your bum back and keeping the weight in your right heel. Keep the right knee over your ankle rather than your toes in the deepest part of the lunge to protect your knees. Ensure the load is distributed more in the glutes and hamstrings than in the quads (b).
- Exhale to engage as you straighten your right leg to press back up.

Safety Considerations

Ensure your beginning stance is wide enough to allow for proper tracking of the front knee. The front knee should be lined up between your first and second toe, but should not move forward over the toes.

Increase Difficulty

- Use dumbbells in both hands or in just one hand to help your body train for uneven loads, such as carrying a car seat.
- When doing this exercise in the first eight weeks postpartum, simply do the base exercise and do not do anything to increase the difficulty.

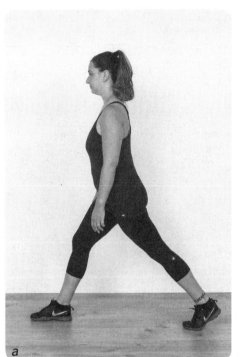 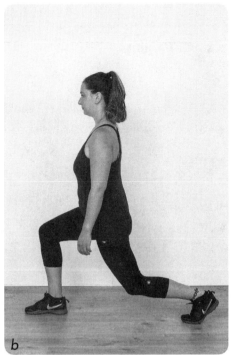

Pelvic Rocking on Stability Ball

Focus and Benefits

- Trains the Core 4 to work as they should with synergy between the diaphragm, pelvic floor, deep abdominals, and multifidus
- Keeps mobility in the pelvis when used during labor
- Releases tension and builds stability in the pelvic floor muscles

Equipment

Stability ball

Description

- Sit on a stability ball with a neutral pelvis.
- Keeping your upper body still, rock and rotate your pelvis: rotate side to side, front to back, in circles, and in figure eights in all directions (a and b).

Safety Considerations

Place the ball next to a wall for stability if needed.

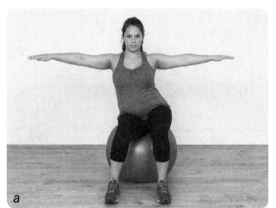
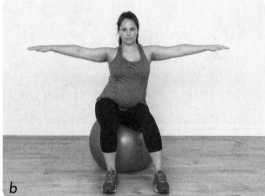

Cat and Cow

Focus and Benefits

- Loads the core against gravity
- Prevents tension patterns from forming in the obliques
- Prepares you for an all-fours position in labor
- Beyond the first eight weeks postpartum, it is a nice gentle exercise to add in to your routine

Equipment

Mat

Description

- Assume a position on all fours with your hands aligned under your shoulders and your knees under your hips and pelvis-width apart.
- Inhale to expand and extend your spine to the cow position (allow your spine to sag down toward the floor) *(a)*.
- Exhale to engage and flex into the cat position (curl your spine toward the ceiling) *(b)*.

Safety Considerations

Avoid this position in the second and third trimesters to minimize added strain on the linea alba in a static front-loaded position (recall from chapter 1 that the linea alba is the connective tissue that connects the two straps of the rectus abdominis at the midline).

Instead, flex and extend your spine gently while standing or seated on a stability ball to reap the benefits of the movement without the additional strain on the connective tissue.

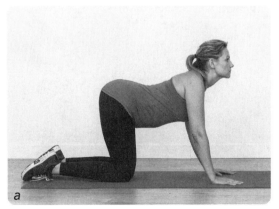
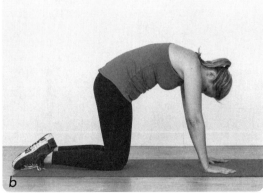

a   b

Side Knee Plank

Focus and Benefits

- Builds strength and endurance in the lateral hip muscles
- Trains the Core 4 to work as they should with synergy between the diaphragm, pelvic floor, deep abdominals, and multifidus
- Prepares you for side-lying positions in labor
- Helps prepare you to progress back to doing full planks

Equipment

Mat

Description

- Sit on your right butt cheek with your knees bent and stacked one on top of the other. Your knees will be in front of you with your heels in line with your glutes.
- Lower your upper body down so you are supporting your weight on your right hip and right elbow. Your spine is in neutral and should not be in contact with the floor. Rest your left arm on your left side.
- Inhale to expand and prepare.
- Exhale to engage, pressing your hips forward until your hips are off the ground and your legs and torso are in a straight line.
- Inhale as you lower your hips back down.

Safety Considerations

Avoid this exercise if it produces any pain or discomfort in your pubic joint.

Increase Difficulty

- Hold the position for 5 to 10 seconds before lowering down.
- Once you are in the pose, lift and lower the top leg to add a dynamic component.

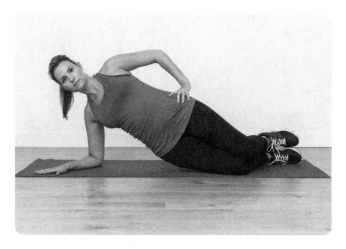

Ball Squeeze Rotation

Focus and Benefits

- Trains the Core 4 to work as they should with synergy between the diaphragm, pelvic floor, deep abdominals, and multifidus
- Prepares you for rotation movements in motherhood
- Incorporates rotation in a gentle way

Equipment

Stability ball or chair and small ball

Description

- Sit on a stability ball or chair with a neutral pelvis.
- Hold a small ball between your hands and reach your arms forward at shoulder height, keeping them straight.
- Inhale to expand and prepare.
- Exhale to engage and squeeze the ball while rotating your upper body to the right. Keep your lower body as still as possible.
- Inhale to expand and release the squeeze while returning to the starting position.
- Repeat, alternating between rotating first to the right or first to the left.

Safety Considerations

Keep your feet planted and your pelvis on the ball and only rotate the upper body.

Increase Difficulty

- Perform the exercise in a standing position.
- Hold a weighted ball or dumbbell in your hands.

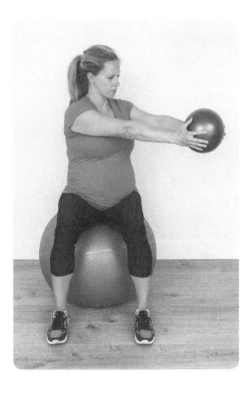

Bird Dog

Focus and Benefits

- Trains the Core 4 to work as they should with synergy between the diaphragm, pelvic floor, deep abdominals, and multifidus
- Focuses on stability and balance

Equipment

Mat

Description

- Assume a position on all fours with your hands aligned under your shoulders and your knees pelvis-width apart under your hips *(a)*.
- Inhale to expand and prepare.
- Exhale to engage and lift your right arm forward and parallel to the floor. At the same time, straighten and lift your left leg backward and parallel to the floor. Keep your arm and leg straight while you hold them up for a few seconds. Your spine and pelvis, should remain neutral, meaning there should be no tipping side to the side, tucking, or overarching *(b)*.
- Inhale to expand as you lower your arm and leg down to the starting position.
- Repeat on the opposite side.

Safety Considerations

Avoid this exercise if you have pain in your pubic joint. Avoid this exercise in the second and third trimesters and do the Standing Bird Dog instead.

Increase Difficulty

Attach a resistance band to your leg and grasp it with the opposite hand so you are using resistance.

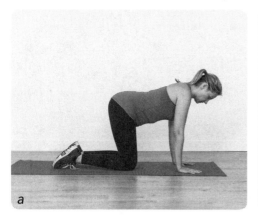

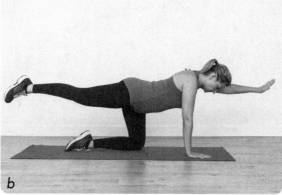

Standing Bird Dog

Focus and Benefits

- Trains the Core 4 to work as they should with synergy between the diaphragm, pelvic floor, deep abdominals, and multifidus
- Focuses on functional movement that involves the core, the upper back, and glutes

Description

- Stand with your feet pelvis-width apart with your arms at your sides.
- Hinge forward at the hips at a 45-degree angle (a).
- Inhale to expand and prepare.
- Exhale to engage and lift the left arm up while extending the right leg back. Create a straight line from your arm, down your torso, to your leg (b).
- Inhale to expand as you lower the arm and leg back to the starting position.
- Repeat on the other side.

Safety Considerations

Raise just your arm or your leg if you are feeling unsteady.

Increase Difficulty

- Hold a lightweight dumbbell with the hand of the arm being raised.
- Perform on a BOSU with the dome up. Note that this is not recommended in the second and third trimesters.

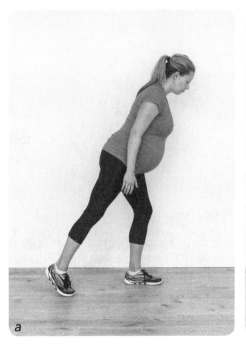
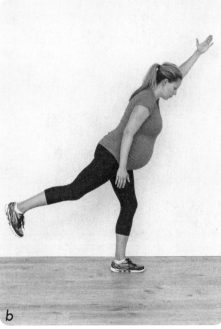

a

b

Crouching Tiger

Focus and Benefits

- Trains the Core 4 to work as they should with synergy between the diaphragm, pelvic floor, deep abdominals, and multifidus
- Works the whole body

Equipment

Mat and small ball or block

Description

- Assume a position on all fours with your hands aligned under your shoulders and your knees under your hips and pelvis-width apart. Place the block or small ball in between your knees *(a)*.
- Inhale to expand and prepare.
- Exhale to engage and lift your knees about two inches off the floor while keeping your pelvis in a neutral position. Feel the tension in the abdominals. You'll be supporting your weight on your hands and toes. Hold for a count of three to five seconds *(b)*.
- Inhale to expand as you lower back down to the starting position.

Safety Considerations

Avoid this position in the second and third trimesters.

Increase Difficulty

- Hold the lifted position of the exercise for 5 to 10 seconds while continuing to breathe.
- Add a crawl (moving forward on your hands and toes) to make the exercise dynamic as opposed to static.

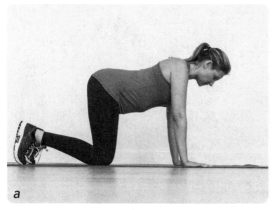
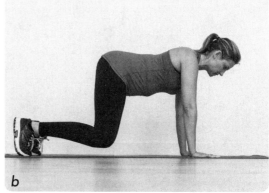

a

b

Front-Loaded Plank

Focus and Benefits
- Targets all the muscles of the core, specifically the rectus abdominis
- Trains the Core 4 to work as they should with synergy between the diaphragm, pelvic floor, deep abdominals, and multifidus

Equipment
Mat

Description
- From a kneeling position, inhale to prepare and exhale to engage. This will create tension across your lower abdominals.
- Lower yourself down onto your elbows, keeping them under your shoulders.
- Inhale to expand and prepare.
- Exhale to engage and then extend one leg back at a time, keeping the pelvis off the mat and the torso parallel to the floor.
- Maintain a neutral spine. Don't sag in the low back.
- Hold for 5 to 10 seconds while taking small breaths

Safety Considerations
- Get into and out of the pose from your knees.
- Don't hold your breath.
- Perform this exercise in the first trimester only. It can be done on an incline or using a wall in later stages to minimize strain on the linea alba.

Increase Difficulty
- Attempt the exercise with straight arms as opposed to resting on your elbows.
- Hold for 10 to 15 seconds.
- Hold on to a BOSU with the dome down instead of having your elbows or hands on the floor.

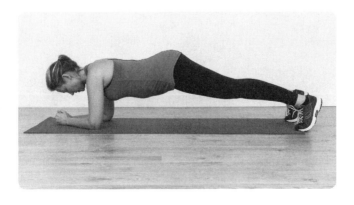

Pallof Press

Focus and Benefits
- Trains the Core 4 to work as they should with synergy between the diaphragm, pelvic floor, deep abdominals, and multifidus both statically and dynamically
- Focuses on stability and balance
- Trains the core, obliques, shoulders, and hips

Equipment
Resistance band

Description
- Attach your resistance band to a stair rail or secure door.
- Stand with your left side facing the door or stair rail and far enough away so there is tension on the resistance band.
- Grip the ends of your resistance band with both hands in a closed fist at your chest (a).
- Inhale to expand.
- Exhale to engage and straighten your arms out in front of you, keeping them at chest height (b).
- The resistance band will want to direct you toward the door or stair rail. You need to resist the desire to rotate while extending and bending the arms.
- Inhale to expand as you return to the starting position.
- Repeat on the opposite side.

Safety Considerations
Start with minimal tension on the resistance band until you are familiar with the movement and do not rotate your spine.

Increase Difficulty
- Use a stronger resistance band.
- Stand farther from the door or stair rail.
- Stand on a BOSU with the dome up (not recommended in the second and third trimester).

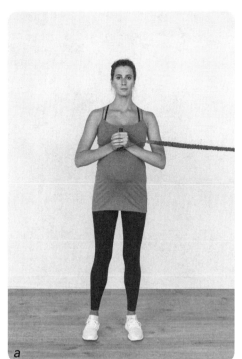 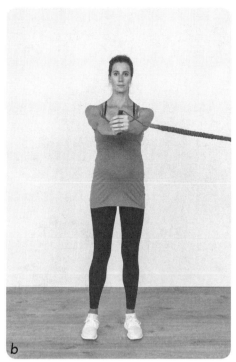

Strength and Endurance for the Upper Body

7

Of all the changes in a pregnant body, the growing belly is the most obvious. Less obvious is what happens to the shoulder girdle and neck during pregnancy. The shoulders begin to round forward, due to both the shifting center of gravity and the larger breasts. The head also starts to jut forward, putting additional strain on the neck. Similar posture changes can also be seen in many people who are not pregnant but who sit for the majority of the day: they have tucked tailbones, flat glutes, weak abdominals, rounded shoulders, and jutting heads—it is becoming an epidemic! Fortunately, the proper stretch and release exercises, coupled with strength training that targets the weak, underused muscles, can prevent or minimize these changes.

CHEST

Generally speaking, the chest is pretty tight in most people. Our days are spent doing tasks that require reaching and bending toward things in front of us. For example, computers and phones are huge contributors to rounded shoulders and tight chest muscles, as are cooking and cleaning. When you add the extra carrying and lifting in pregnancy and motherhood, the rounding and tightness can be exacerbated. The breasts are typically larger and heavier, there are biomechanical changes in the pregnant body that alter optimal alignment, and once the baby is born there is the influence of breastfeeding and baby-carrying as well. Just because a muscle is tight does not mean it is strong, so it is still important to strengthen this area of the body. Just be sure to balance the strengthening out with a lot of stretching and release work for the chest and shoulders.

Wall Push-Up

Focus and Benefits

Push-ups are a great exercise for the chest, shoulders, and triceps—even the core—but as the pregnancy advances, full front-loaded push-ups are not ideal given the additional strain on the abdominal wall. Using a wall allows the body to be more upright so there is still some loading to the abdominal wall (a good thing) without full straining.

Equipment

Wall

Description

- Stand in front of a wall with your hands on the wall at shoulder height.
- Take one step back so your body is on a slight forward angle and arms are parallel to the floor (a).
- Inhale to expand as you lower your chest to the wall (b).
- Exhale to engage as you press away from the wall.

Safety Considerations

Start with a small step away from the wall until you build up endurance and comfort in the exercise.

Increase Difficulty

- Try lifting one foot off the ground and keep it off as you do the push-up.
- Step back a little further from the wall.

Change It Up

Push-ups are typically done with both hands on the ground. Extreme boot camp style workouts will often show one-arm versions, which are very tough! In pregnancy, we recommend wall push-ups and we describe them being done with both hands on the wall. You can however, add a little boot camp in there and try some one-arm versions to mix it up a bit. Training one side at a time gives a different challenge to the arms, chest, and core!

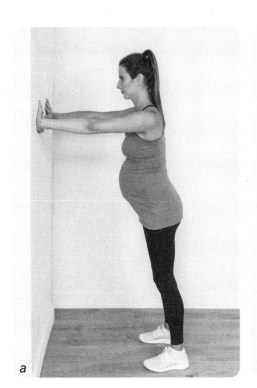 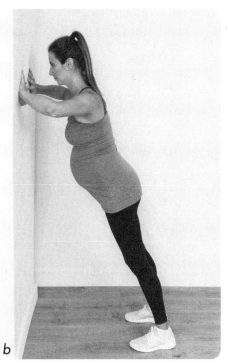

Chest Press With Band

Focus and Benefits

Using a band for a chest press is a nice way to train. The band is lightweight, so you can take it with you on the go. It trains the muscles differently than a machine or dumbbell. Variety is key! Doing this exercise while standing adds in some great core work, too.

Equipment

Resistance band

Description

- Wrap the resistance band around a pole or bannister at chest height.
- Turn around so your back is facing the pole or bannister and grasp one end of the band in each hand.
- Raise your hands and elbows to shoulder height with your palms faced down toward the floor.
- Step forward with one leg and lean slightly forward to create desired tension while inhaling to expand your chest *(a)*.
- As you exhale to engage, extend your arms forward in front of your chest *(b)*.

Safety Considerations

- Ensure the pole or bannister is sturdy.
- Resist the band on the way back to the start instead of allowing the band to snap back.

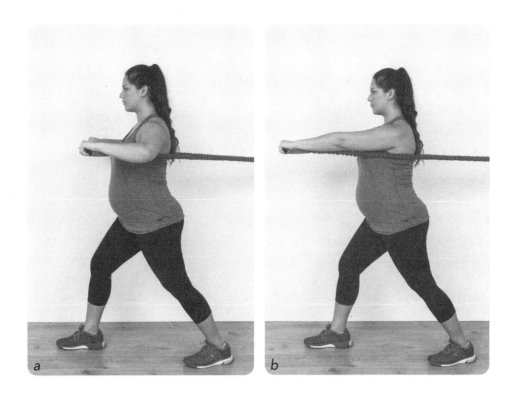

a

b

Suspension devices are a great tool for chest work. Using the door attachment, secure your device, turn so your back is facing the door, then take both handles in your hands. With your arms extended in front of you, walk your feet back toward the door until your body is on a slight forward angle, then perform a standing push-up. As your pregnancy progresses, reduce the angle or choose wall push-ups instead.

Walkover Push-Up on BOSU

Focus and Benefits

Working the body dynamically trains you for the demands of motherhood while also building great arms and shoulders!

Equipment

BOSU and mat

Description

- Kneel on the floor with a neutral pelvis in front of a BOSU with the dome side up.
- Inhale to expand and as you exhale, engage your pelvic floor to create tension across the lower abdominals.
- Maintain this tension and bend over to place one hand on the floor and the other on the center (top) of the dome.
- Scoot your knees back, and drop your hips until your spine is in a neutral position and your chest is level with the top of the dome of the BOSU *(a)*.
- Inhale as you bend and bring your chest toward the floor on one side of the BOSU *(b)*.
- Exhale to engage and push up as you walk your hands across the top of the dome and switch sides.

Safety Considerations

If you feel any pressure in your pelvic floor or pain in the low back, omit this exercise and stick with the wall push-ups.

Increase Difficulty

You can increase the number of reps, slow your movement down, or you can go up on your toes to make this more challenging. This is not recommended in the second or third trimesters.

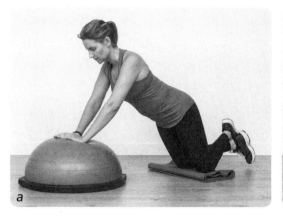
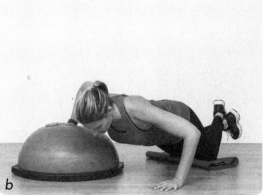

a

b

Kneeling Ball Squeeze

Focus and Benefits

Why train just the chest? Adding in some amazing core work really ups the ante on this exercise!

Equipment

BOSU and stability ball

Description

- Kneel on top of the dome of a BOSU, either resting the toes of both feet on the floor or lifting one foot or both feet up off the floor to increase intensity.
- Hold a stability ball in front of you with one hand on either side and lift it up so it is shoulder height, elbows out to the sides and your thighs are vertical.
- Inhale to expand, and as you exhale to engage, squeeze the ball.

Safety Considerations

If kneeling on the BOSU feels unstable, you can kneel on a mat and do the ball squeezes.

Increase Difficulty

Increase the number of reps you do to increase the challenge.

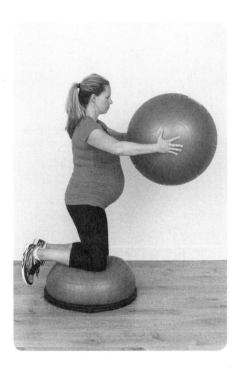

Incline Chest Press on Bench

Focus and Benefits

When you add different angles, you target different aspects of the muscle. The incline also gets a little more into the front of the shoulders.

Equipment

Adjustable bench and dumbbells

Description

- Adjust the back of the bench to an incline position and sit on the bench with your legs to one side.
- Hold a dumbbell in each hand close to you, lean to the side until you are side-lying on the bench, then roll onto your back. This helps protect the abdominal wall.
- Once on your back, allow the elbows to bend so the dumbbells can be pushed up *(a)*.
- Inhale to expand and prepare.
- Exhale to engage as you press the weights up over your chest *(b)*.

Safety Considerations

If rolling over on the bench feels awkward or unstable, choose another exercise.

Increase Difficulty

Use a heavier weight and slow the speed of your reps to increase the challenge.

Change It Up

Using a bench is common for supine chest work in fitness. You can also use the floor or, if you feel you want a little more variety, a stability ball. The best way to get into a table-top position on a stability ball when you are pregnant is to place the ball on the floor in front of a wall, then sit on your bum with your back against the ball. Bend your head back until your head and back are in contact with the ball, and then push your hips up and roll your torso to the top of the ball until your pelvis is in a neutral position and your torso is parallel to the ground. Ideally you have your weights in your hands already or you have someone there to hand the weights to you. However, you should practice getting into and out of the table-top position on the ball before using weights. Once you have the movement down, you can grab your dumbbells.

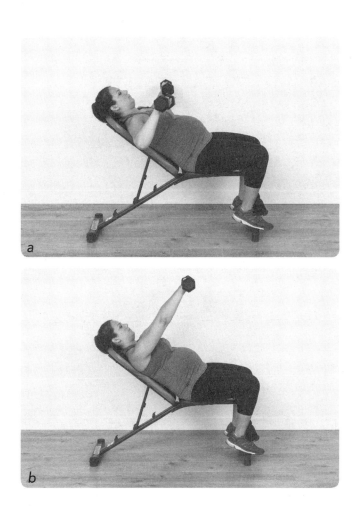

Push-Up

Focus and Benefits

The push-up is often categorized as a chest exercise but is really a full-body exercise that is great for the shoulders and chest.

Equipment

Mat

Description

- Sit on your knees in an upright position.
- Inhale to expand, then, as you exhale, create tension across your lower abdominals.
- Maintain that tension and go into a push-up position with your knees on the floor and your hands under your shoulders *(a)*.
- Inhale to expand as you lower your chest to the floor *(b)*.
- Exhale to engage and press back up.

Safety Considerations

- This is recommended for the first trimester only.
- Ensure your low back does not sag or overarch. Maintain a neutral pelvis.

Increase Difficulty

Extend the legs straight so you are in a full push-up position for an added challenge.

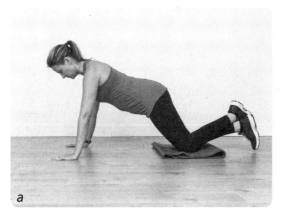

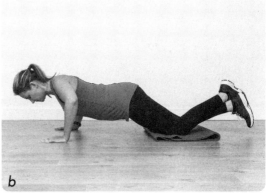

BACK

Back pain is becoming increasingly common and pregnancy can certainly bring on back pain if you haven't experienced it until now. A 2008 study found the pregnant women experience more back pain than non-pregnant women (Smith, Russell, and Hodges 2008). Hormonal changes, biomechanical changes, alignment changes, heavier breasts, shifting center of gravity—these can all contribute to more aches and pains in the back. Awareness, movement, and release work can all help relieve and even avoid back pain.

One-Arm Reverse Fly

Focus and Benefits
With its focus on the upper back and shoulders, this is a great posture-improving exercise.

Equipment
Resistance band

Description
- Stand with a neutral pelvis with the resistance band under your let foot and hold the band in your right hand.
- While holding the band, cross the right hand over to the left hip *(a)*.
- Inhale to expand and prepare.
- Exhale to engage and pull the band out across the front of your body to the right while keeping your arm straight *(b)*.
- Squeeze your right shoulder blade without rotating your spine.
- Inhale to expand as you lower your arm back to the starting position.
- Repeat on the other side.

Safety Considerations
Ensure your band is securely fastened.

Increase Difficulty
- You can do both arms at the same time by standing with both feet on the center of the band and having two ends to use.
- Increase the number of reps.
- Use a thicker band with more resistance.

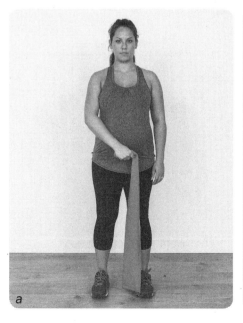
a

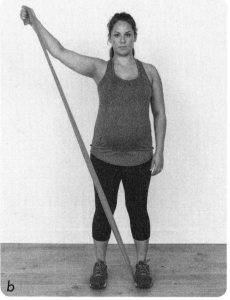
b

Seated Back Row

Focus and Benefits

Everyone should do row exercises, especially pregnant women and new moms. This exercise will help minimize aches and pains and ensure the upper back is ready to support breastfeeding and baby-carrying.

Equipment

Stability ball or bench and resistance band

Description

- Sit on a stability ball or bench with the resistance band looped around a bannister or attached to a door or other stable object.
- Grasp the ends of the band in each hand, facing the bannister or door with arms extended out front *(a)*.
- Inhale to expand and prepare.
- Exhale to engage as you pull the band toward you, driving your elbows back and squeezing your shoulder blades together *(b)*.
- Keep your elbows in close to the sides of your body.

Safety Considerations

Ensure you are sitting with a neutral pelvis and that the movement is from the arms, not the body.

Increase Difficulty

- Perform the exercise from a standing position.
- Choose a thicker resistance band for added resistance.
- Increase the number of reps.

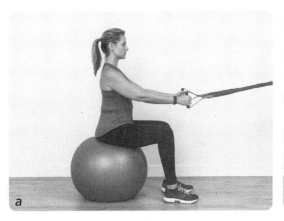
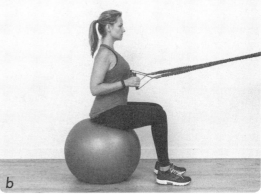

a

b

Standing Shoulder Retraction

Focus and Benefits

Keeping the upper back strong will help minimize rounding of your shoulders. This exercise is very targeted and gets the deep muscles.

Equipment

Resistance band

Description

- Stand with one end of the band in each hand and your arms straight out in front so that there is enough tension to keep the band taught but not tight (a).
- Inhale to expand and prepare.
- Exhale to engage and squeeze your shoulder blades together while keeping your arms straight (b).

Safety Considerations

Ensure you are standing with a neutral pelvis.

Increase Difficulty

- Choose a thicker band for more resistance.
- Increase the number of reps.
- Hold your hands closer together on the band.

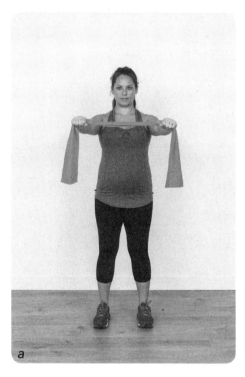
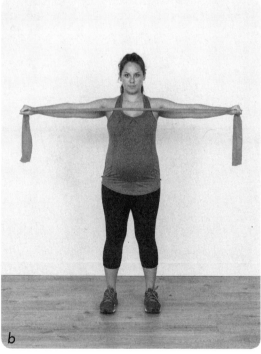

a

b

Seated Lat Pulldown

Focus and Benefits

The focus of this exercise is the lats and it is done in an upright position, which changes things up from the one-arm row.

Equipment

Stability ball or bench and resistance band

Description

- Sit on a stability ball or bench.
- Hold the resistance band in both hands about shoulder-width apart with your arms straight up over your head (a).
- Exhale to engage and pull your arms apart from each other while bringing the band down to the chest, keeping your arms straight (b).

Safety Considerations

- Make sure you sit with a neutral pelvis.
- Do not lock your elbows.

Increase Difficulty

- Choose a thicker resistance band for added difficulty.
- Increase the number of reps.
- Try lifting one foot slightly off the floor while ensuring you maintain a neutral pelvis.

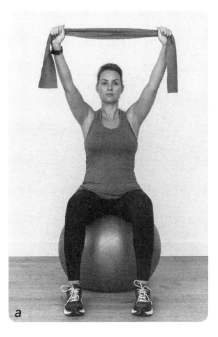
a

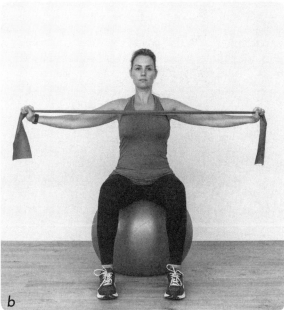
b

One-Arm Bent-Over Row

Focus and Benefits

This exercise focuses on muscles in the shoulder and the back as well as the biceps.

Equipment

Bench and dumbbell

Description

- Stand tall with a neutral pelvis holding one dumbbell in your left hand.
- Inhale to expand and as you exhale, create tension across your lower abdominals.
- Maintain that tension as you place your right knee on a bench. At the same time, bend down and place your right hand firmly on the bench, while keeping your hand under your right shoulder for added support.
- Keep your pelvis in a neutral position.
- Let the weight in the left hand hang freely toward the floor without dropping the shoulder (a).
- Inhale to expand. Then, exhale to engage and drive the elbow back and up and squeeze the shoulder blade (b).
- Switch sides.

Safety Considerations

- Keep the body still and avoid rotating as you lift the dumbbell.
- Ensure your low back does not sag or overarch.

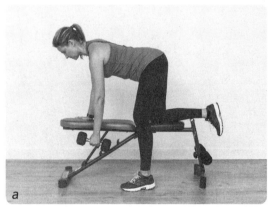
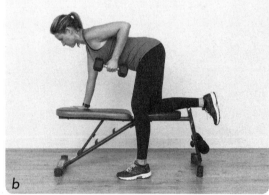

Increase Difficulty

- Increase the number of reps.
- Grab a heavier dumbbell.
- Do both arms at the same time while standing with hips flexed in a bent-over position.

CHALLENGE YOURSELF Using a stability ball can bring other muscles into a more focused exercise. When doing a one-arm row, try using a stability ball instead of a bench as your base of support. You can keep both knees on the ground and place the support hand on the ball. The subtle movements of the unstable ball mean you need to work at keeping the ball still while also performing the exercise. For even more challenge, try putting one knee on the ball, which decreases your base of support and increases the challenge to your balance and core.

Bent-Over Reverse Fly

Focus and Benefits

This exercise provides some challenge to the core while working the backs of the shoulders.

Equipment

Dumbbells

Description

- Stand with a neutral pelvis, holding a dumbbell in each hand.
- Bend forward from the hips to approximately 45 degrees and let the dumbbells hang freely toward the floor without dropping the shoulders *(a)*.
- Inhale to expand and prepare.
- Exhale to engage and then, keeping arms straight, lift the weights to the sides and up toward the ceiling while squeezing the shoulder blades *(b)*.

Safety Considerations

- If you feel any pressure in your pelvis or pain in your back, choose a resistance band and do this exercise from an upright position.
- Don't lock your elbows.

Increase Difficulty

- Choose heavier dumbbells for added resistance.
- Increase the number of reps.

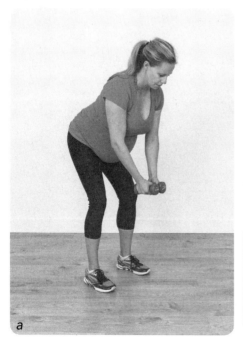
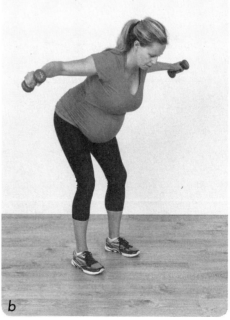

a   b

Upright Row

Focus and Benefits

You will be doing a lot of lifting and having strong shoulders will help. This exercise really targets the shoulders.

Equipment

Dumbbells

Description

- Stand with a neutral pelvis and hold a dumbbell in each hand in front of your belly with palms resting on the front of your thighs *(a)*.
- Inhale to expand and prepare.
- Exhale to engage as you lead with the elbows and lift the dumbbells to chest height *(b)*.

Safety Considerations

- As your belly gets bigger you may wish to switch to a resistance band so as not to hit your belly with the dumbbells.
- If you feel any discomfort you can stand in a staggered stance.

Increase Difficulty

- Choose heavier dumbbells for added resistance.
- Increase the number of reps.

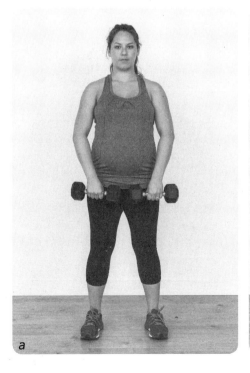
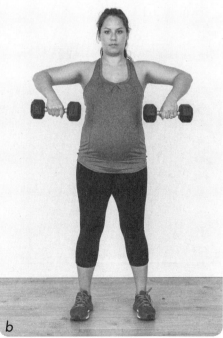

a

b

Standing One-Arm Back Row

Focus and Benefits

This is a great exercise for the lats and biceps and also gives a nice stretch to the legs for an added benefit.

Equipment

Dumbbell

Description

- Stand tall with a neutral pelvis, holding a dumbbell in your left hand at your side.
- Step forward with your right leg and place your right hand on the front of your right thigh.
- Extend the left leg behind you and bend your right leg.
- Let the dumbbell hang freely toward the floor without dropping your shoulder (a).
- Inhale to expand.
- Exhale to engage and drive the elbow back, squeezing the shoulder blade (b).
- Switch sides.

Safety Considerations

If you feel unsteady, you can place your support hand on the back of a chair instead of your thigh.

Increase Difficulty

- Choose a heavier dumbbell for increased resistance.
- Increase the number of reps.

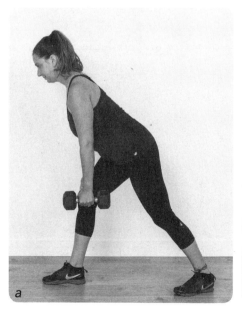
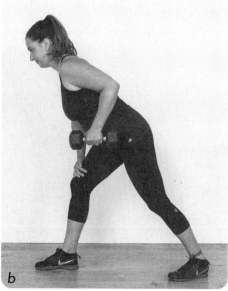

a

b

Squat and Back Row

Focus and Benefits
Compound exercises increase the challenge and make your workouts more efficient because you are working more than one major muscle group at a time. Here we target the back while also getting some squats in.

Equipment
Resistance band

Description
- Wrap the resistance band around a post or bannister.
- Face the bannister and grab one end of the band with each hand.
- Walk backward until you reach the desired resistance, then stand tall with a neutral pelvis.
- Inhale to expand as you extend your arms forward and sit back into a squat *(a)*.
- Exhale to engage as you return to standing while driving your elbows back and squeezing your shoulder blades *(b)*.

Safety Considerations
Ensure you maintain a neutral pelvis throughout the squat.

Increase Difficulty
- Choose a thicker resistance band for added resistance.
- Increase the number of reps.

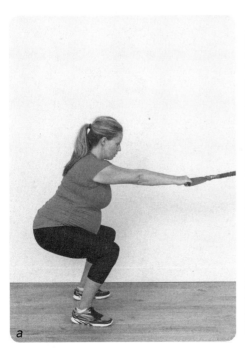
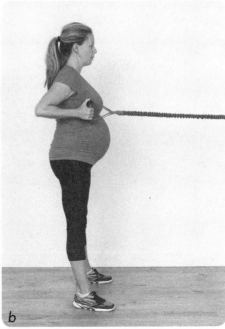

Standing Lat Pulldown

Focus and Benefits

This is a great exercise for the back, which is a little more challenging than the seated lat pulldown.

Equipment

Resistance band

Description

- Stand with feet pelvis-width apart and one end of the resistance band in each hand about shoulder-width apart.
- Inhale to expand, reaching your arms straight up over your head *(a)*.
- Exhale to engage and pull arms apart from each other while bringing the band to the chest, keeping arms straight *(b)*.

Safety Considerations

- If you feel unsteady or have any pressure in your pelvis, stagger your stance so that you have one foot out front and one back, similar to a lunge but with a narrower stance.
- Don't lock your elbows.

Increase Difficulty

- Increase the resistance of the band for a greater challenge.
- Increase the number of reps.

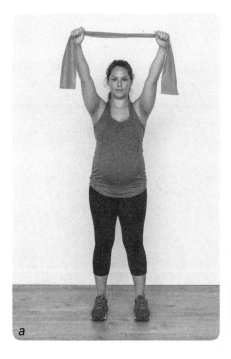
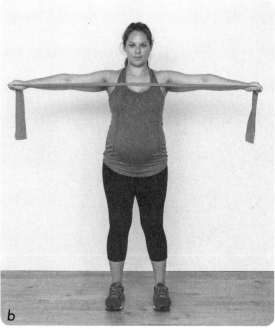

a

b

Lunge and One-Arm Row

Focus and Benefits

This exercise is another compound movement to work on strength, coordination, and endurance.

Equipment

Resistance band

Description

- Wrap resistance band around a post or bannister.
- Hold both ends of the band with the right hand.
- Step back to desired resistance and extend your right leg behind you.
- Inhale to expand as you bend your right leg and lower into a lunge position (a).
- Exhale to engage as you press up with your left leg and drive the right elbow back (b).
- Squeeze your right shoulder blade.
- Repeat on the other side.

Safety Considerations

If you feel unsteady you can decrease the distance between your legs for more support.

Increase Difficulty

- Increase the thickness of the resistance band for more resistance.
- Increase the number of reps.
- Do a row with both hands instead of one at a time.

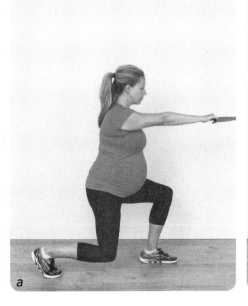

a

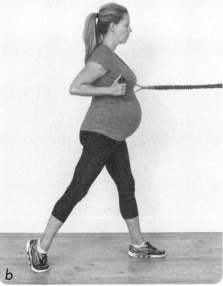

b

ARMS

Your arms will be carrying a lot more than they are used to once your baby is born. They will be holding your baby, lifting and carrying loads of laundry, lifting the car seat or stroller into and out of the car, and pushing the stroller on walks. Let's build up their strength and endurance before your baby arrives.

Preacher Curl

Focus and Benefits

Preacher curls targets the biceps and remove the opportunity to use your body weight for help.

Equipment

Dumbbells

Description

- Kneel on the floor with a stability ball in front of you.
- Hold dumbbells in your hands and place the backs of your arms on the ball with your arms extended (a).
- Inhale to expand and prepare.
- Exhale to engage and curl the dumbbells up toward the shoulders (b).

Safety Considerations

- Ensure the wrists stay in neutral during the lift.
- Don't lock your elbows on the extension part of the exercise.

Increase Difficulty

- Increase the weight of the dumbbells for an added challenge.
- Increase the number of reps.

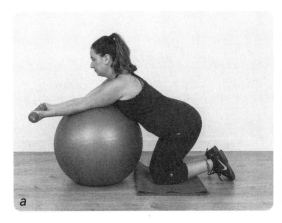
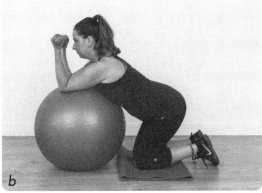

a

b

Standing Biceps Curl

Focus and Benefits

This exercise focuses on your biceps, which help you lift.

Equipment

Dumbbells

Description

- Stand with feet pelvis-width apart and your pelvis in a neutral position.
- Hold a dumbbell in each hand with your arms at your sides and palms facing out to the front (a).
- Inhale to expand and prepare.
- Exhale to engage and bend your elbows while bringing the dumbbells toward your shoulders (b).

Safety Considerations

Ensure you use your arms and do not arch your back or bend backward to try to help lift the dumbbells.

Increase Difficulty

- Increase the weight of the dumbbells for greater resistance.
- Increase the number of reps.
- Try standing on one leg while performing the exercise.

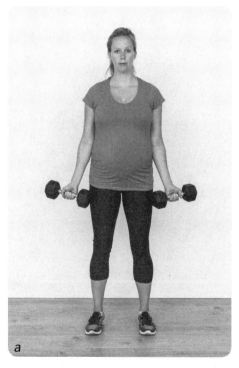
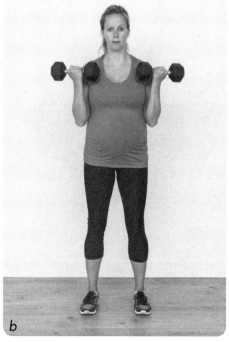

a

b

Change It Up

Doing regular biceps curls can be a little boring, so why not get more bang for your buck in less time? Try some supersets (you can do this with any set of exercises). Do a set of standard biceps curls and then right away, with no rest, do a set of hammer curls. Another method to try would be to use different ranges of motion. Do five reps from the bottom of the curl but lifting only halfway up. Then do five reps starting from halfway to all the way up. Then finish with five full reps from bottom to top. Your biceps will definitely be speaking to you after that!

Incline Biceps Curl on Bench

Focus and Benefits
Lying back on the bench targets the biceps at a new angle for a different challenge.

Equipment
Adjustable bench and dumbbells

Description
- Adjust the bench to a 45-degree angle. Holding a dumbbell in each hand, sit on the bench with both legs on one side.
- Lean sideways and lower onto the bench into a side-lying position, then roll onto your back.
- Let the dumbbells hang freely toward the floor (a).
- Inhale to expand and prepare.
- Exhale to engage and curl the dumbbells up toward your shoulders (b).

Safety Considerations
- Make sure you get into and out of the position by rolling onto your side first.
- Bend at the elbows only. Do not move the shoulder joint during the lift.

Increase Difficulty
Use heavier dumbbells for greater resistance.

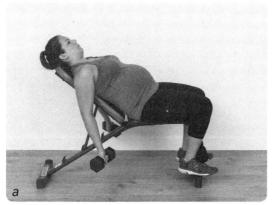
a

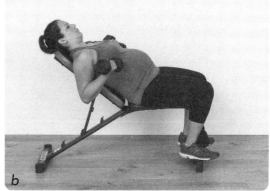
b

Standing Hammer Curl

Focus and Benefits
A slight turn of the arms targets the biceps from a different angle—because life isn't always one direction.

Equipment
Dumbbells

Description
- Stand with feet pelvis-width apart and a neutral pelvis.
- Hold a dumbbell in each hand with your arms at your sides, palms facing in toward your body (a).
- Inhale to expand and prepare.
- Exhale to engage and bend your elbows while bringing the dumbbells toward your shoulders (b).

Safety Considerations
Ensure wrists stay neutral.

Increase Difficulty
- Grab heavier weights for more challenge.
- Increase the number of reps.
- Stand on one leg and complete the hammer curls.

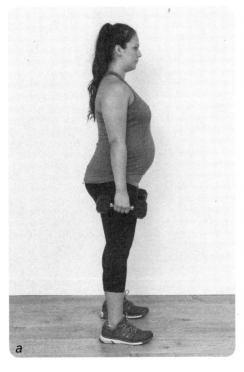

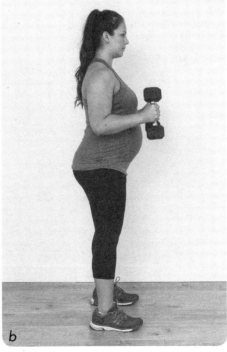

a

b

Barbell Biceps Curl

Focus and Benefits

This is a classic. As your belly gets bigger, it may work better to use dumbbells, but the barbell biceps curl is a tried and true exercise for the arms.

Equipment

Barbell

Description

- Stand with feet pelvis-width apart and with a neutral pelvis.
- Hold a barbell in front of your body with an underhand grip (palms facing forward when barbell is lowered) and with the hands shoulder-width apart (a).
- Inhale to expand and prepare.
- Exhale to engage and bend your elbows while bringing the barbell toward your shoulders; be sure to keeps your wrists neutral (b).

Safety Considerations

- Ensure the barbell does not hit your belly.
- Keep the weight in a range where you can lift without arching your back.

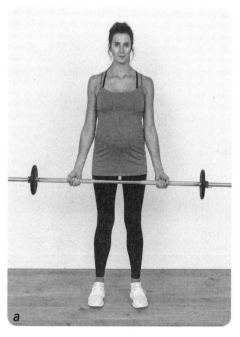
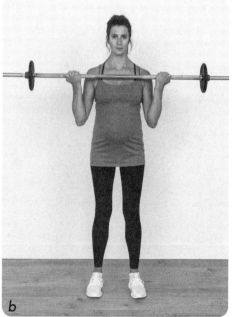

a
b

CHALLENGE YOURSELF Combining a barbell biceps curl with a deadlift is a great way to get your heart rate up and work on two body parts—legs and arms. It will also get you ready for picking up laundry baskets and children.

Seated Biceps Curl

Focus and Benefits

Sometimes standing just seems tough, especially as the pregnancy progresses. When you are feeling a bit tired but still want to get some resistance training in, do your biceps curls seated.

Equipment

Stability ball or bench and dumbbells

Description

- Sit on a stability ball or bench with a neutral pelvis.
- Hold a dumbbell in each hand with your arms at your sides and palms facing forward (for a regular curl) or inward toward your body (for a hammer curl).
- Inhale to expand and prepare *(a)*.
- Exhale to engage and curl the weights up toward your shoulders *(b)*.

Safety Considerations

If you feel unsteady on the ball, use a bench or wedge your ball into a corner.

Increase Difficulty

- Increase the weight for more challenge.
- Increase the number of reps.
- Try completing the exercise with one foot slightly off the ground.

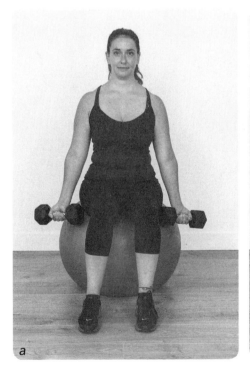

a

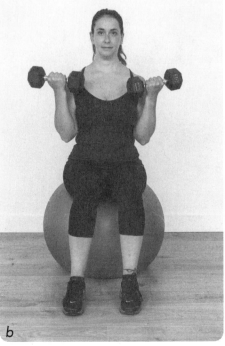

b

Hammer Curl and Shoulder Press

Focus and Benefits

Adding a shoulder press to a hammer curl means you'll be working two sets of muscles in one exercise, making it more efficient and effective.

Equipment

Dumbbells

Description

- Stand with feet pelvis-width apart and a neutral pelvis.
- Hold a dumbbell in each hand with your arms by your sides and palms facing your body.
- Inhale to expand and prepare.
- Exhale to engage and curl the dumbbells toward your shoulders (a).
- Pause at the top while you inhale to expand again.
- Exhale to engage and press the dumbbells up over your head (b).

Safety Considerations

Ensure the weight is manageable and allows you to complete the movement without arching your back.

Increase Difficulty

- Grab a heavier set of dumbbells for a greater challenge.
- Increase the number of reps.
- Try with one foot lifted off the ground.

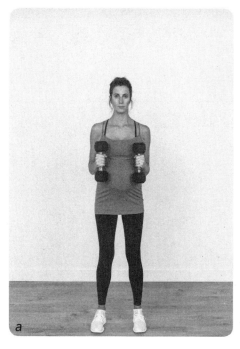
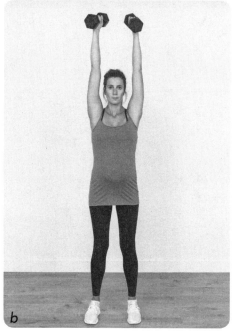

a

b

Kneeling Biceps Curl on BOSU

Focus and Benefits

Adding some instability to your base of support brings in other parts of the body while still focusing on the biceps.

Equipment

BOSU and dumbbells

Description

- Kneel on the dome of a BOSU, either lifting the toes or leaving them on the floor for stability.
- Hold a dumbbell in each hand with your arms at your sides and palms facing front *(a)*.
- Inhale to prepare.
- Exhale to engage as you bend your elbows and bring the weights toward your shoulders *(b)*.

Safety Considerations

If you feel unsteady, keep your toes on the ground.

Increase Difficulty

Add a shoulder press after the biceps curl to increase the challenge.

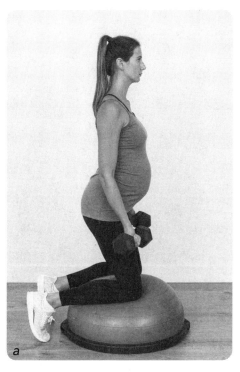
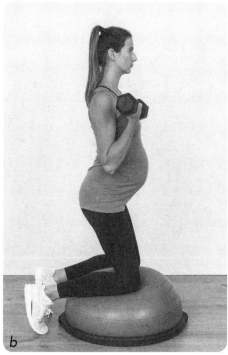

a

b

Lunge With Biceps Curl

Focus and Benefits

Bringing some dynamic movement into the biceps curl to work on coordination is a great way to make your workouts more efficient.

Equipment

Dumbbells

Description

- Stand tall with feet pelvis-width apart and a neutral pelvis.
- Hold a dumbbell in each hand with your arms at your sides and palms facing front.
- Extend one leg behind you keeping the heel off the floor.
- Inhale to prepare as you bend the back leg until you are in a lunge stance and both legs are bent approximately 90 degrees (a).
- Exhale to engage as you straighten your front leg to press back up. At the same time, bend at the elbows and bring the dumbbells toward the shoulders (b).

Safety Considerations

If you feel unsteady you can hold on to the back of a chair with one hand and do the biceps curl with only the free hand.

Increase Difficulty

- Grab heavier dumbbells for greater resistance.
- Increase the number of reps.
- Lengthen your lunge stance for more challenge.

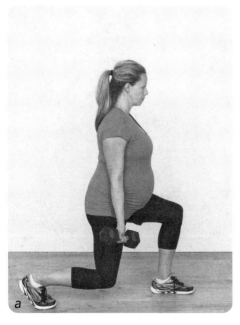 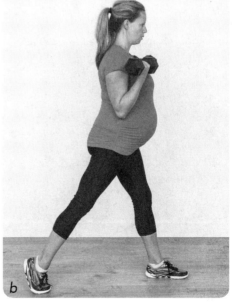

Standing Biceps Curl on BOSU

Focus and Benefits

The instability of the BOSU offers increased challenge for your core and entire body as you do your biceps curls.

Equipment

BOSU and dumbbells

Description

- Stand on the dome of a BOSU with your feet comfortably apart and a neutral pelvis.
- Hold a dumbbell in each hand with your arms at your sides and palms facing front *(a)*.
- Inhale to prepare.
- Exhale to engage as you bend at the elbows and bring the weights toward your shoulders *(b)*.

Safety Considerations

If standing on the BOSU makes you feel too unstable, especially in the later months of pregnancy, opt for standing biceps curls.

Increase Difficulty

- Heavier dumbbells will increase the resistance.
- Increase the number of reps.

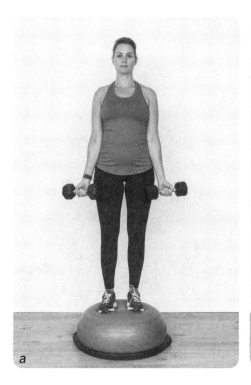
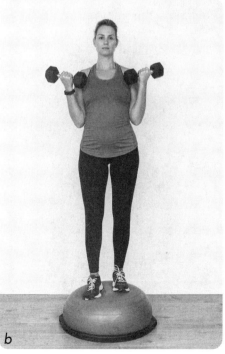

a

b

Concentration Curl

Focus and Benefits

This exercise is a great way to target the biceps while ensuring that you have a stable base of support.

Equipment

Chair or stability ball and dumbbell

Description

- Sit tall on a chair or stability ball with a neutral pelvis and your feet spread comfortably apart.
- Hold the dumbbell in your right hand.
- Hinge forward at the hips and rest the back of your right arm on the inside of the right thigh *(a)*.
- Place your left hand on your left thigh for support.
- Inhale to prepare.
- Exhale to engage as you bend the right arm at the elbow and bring the dumbbell toward the shoulder *(b)*.

Safety Considerations

- Keep the wrist neutral.
- Maintain neutral posture and don't round your shoulders.

Increase Difficulty

- Grab a heavier dumbbell for a greater challenge.
- Increase the number of reps.

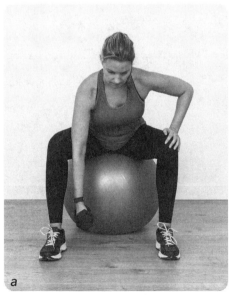

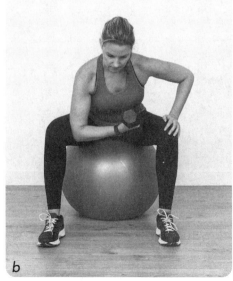

Ball Squat With Biceps Curl

Focus and Benefits

Deep squats are great preparation for labor. Having a stability ball behind you gives you support while you gain the benefits from squats. Why not add a biceps curl while you are doing your squats?

Equipment

Stability ball and dumbbells

Description

- Grab a dumbbell in each hand and then place a stability ball against the wall.
- Stand with the ball in the small of your back and with your feet pelvis width apart and slightly out in front.
- Let the back of your arms rest on either side of the ball with palms facing out .
- Inhale to expand as you lower down into a squat *(a)*.
- Exhale to engage as you stand up from the squat and bend the elbows and bring the dumbbells toward your shoulders *(b)*.

Safety Considerations

If you feel any pressure on your knees, simply return to any of the other biceps curl exercises.

Increase Difficulty

- Grab a heavier set of dumbbells to increase the challenge.
- Increase the number of reps.

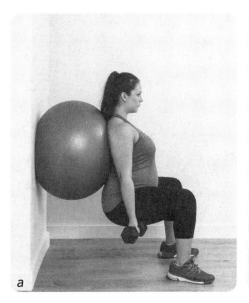

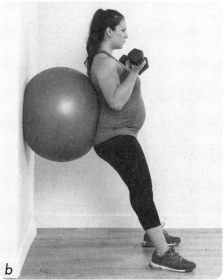

Skull Crusher

Focus and Benefits
The name is a bit scary but this is a great exercise to target the triceps.

Equipment
Adjustable bench or mat on the floor and dumbbells

Description
- Lie on the bench (or mat) with your knees bent and your feet on the floor.
- Hold a dumbbell in each hand with your arms at your sides and your elbows bent.
- Inhale to prepare.
- Exhale to engage and press your arms straight up over your shoulders toward the ceiling (a).
- Inhale to expand and bend your elbows, allowing the dumbbells to lower toward your ears (b).
- Keep your shoulders stationary and your arms parallel.

Safety Considerations
- Ensure you have a good grip to avoid dropping the weights.
- If you feel unstable on the bench or have a hard time rolling over, do the exercise on the floor.
- Once you hit 20 weeks gestation, adjust the bench to an incline position if you feel uncomfortable flat on your back.

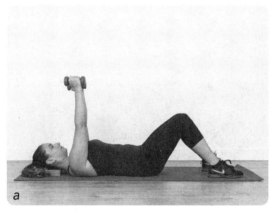 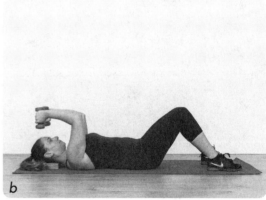

a

b

Triceps Kickback

Focus and Benefits

This exercise works the triceps, which help with push movements and also give the arms nice shape.

Equipment

Bench and dumbbell

Description

- Stand tall beside the bench and hold a dumbbell in your left hand.
- Inhale to prepare and as you exhale, create tension along your lower abdominals.
- Place your right knee on the bench and the right hand under the shoulder. Your left foot is on the floor beside the bench.
- Find your neutral pelvis position.
- Bend your right elbow so the dumbbell is close to your chest and your palm is facing in toward your body (a).
- Inhale to prepare.
- Exhale to engage and extend your right arm back as you squeeze your triceps (b).
- Repeat on the other side.

Safety Considerations

Ensure the weight is light enough that you can fully extend your arm.

Increase Difficulty

- Increase the weight for more challenge.
- Increase the number of reps.

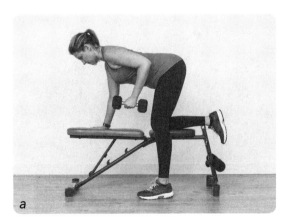
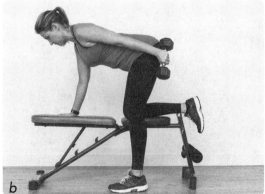

Triceps Press With Stability Ball

Focus and Benefits

This is similar to a push-up but by keeping the elbows pointed toward the floor, you really target the triceps.

Equipment

Stability ball

Description

- Stand about arms' length away from a wall. Place a stability ball against the wall with the top of the ball at eye level.
- Place your hands on the front of the ball with fingers pointed toward the ceiling and elbows pointed toward the floor.
- Keep the arms parallel throughout the exercise
- Extend your arms and step back so you are leaning into the ball (a).
- Maintain a neutral pelvis position.
- Inhale to expand as you bend the elbows and allow your upper body to lean in closer to the ball (b).
- Exhale to engage as you press back to starting position.

Safety Considerations

- If you feel unsteady, wedge the ball into a corner.
- This exercise can also be done without the ball, using just the wall.

Increase Difficulty

Step back farther away from the ball to increase the lean for a greater challenge.

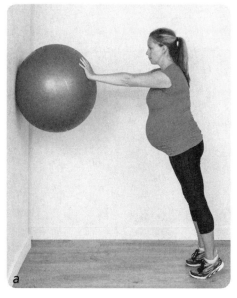 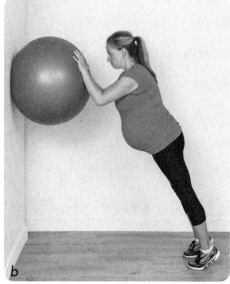

Skull Crusher on Stability Ball

Focus and Benefits

This exercise is similar to the skull crusher you did on the bench or floor, but the ball adds an element of instability for a greater challenge.

Equipment

Stability ball and dumbbells

Description

- Place a stability ball on the floor.
- Place a dumbbell on the floor on either side of you and sit with your back pressing into the stability ball.
- Grab the dumbbells and bend your elbows with your arms at your sides. Lean back, putting your head on the ball and lifting your bum up.
- Walk your feet out until your torso is close to parallel to the floor, then extend and straighten both arms toward the ceiling (a).
- Inhale to expand as you bend at the elbows and bring the weights toward your ears, keeping your arms parallel to each other (b).
- Exhale to engage as you straighten both arms over your head.

Safety Considerations

If the ball feels unstable, wedge it into a corner, place it against a wall, or stick with the bench or floor option.

Increase Difficulty

- Use a heavier set of dumbbells.
- Increase the number of reps.

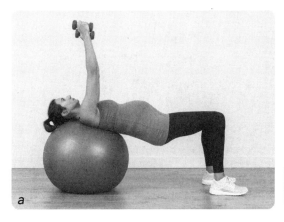
a

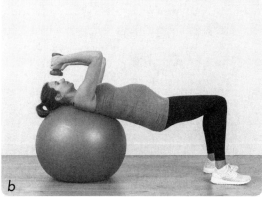
b

Focus and Benefits

While resistance-band training offers a nice smooth movement, dumbbells offer a bit more challenge given the tiny micro-movements they demand of your muscles to stabilize.

Equipment

Bench or stability ball and dumbbell

Description

- Sit tall on a bench or ball with a neutral pelvis and hold one dumbbell with both hands in front of your chest.
- Extend and straighten both arms to lift the dumbbell over your head with elbows pointed forward and beside your ears.
- Inhale to expand as you bend both elbows to lower the dumbbell behind your head *(a)*.
- Exhale to engage as you straighten the arms and raise the dumbbell back up overhead *(b)*.

Safety Considerations

- Ensure you don't lean back or arch your back as you press the dumbbell up.
- Keep your shoulders and neck relaxed.

Increase Difficulty

- Grab a heavier dumbbell for a greater challenge.
- Increase the number of reps.

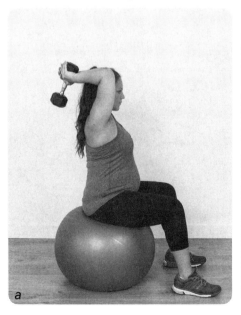
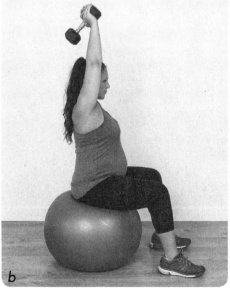

Side-Lying Triceps Press-Up

Focus and Benefits

Exercises that can be done without equipment are always good because they can be done anywhere and they use your own body weight in functional movements.

Equipment

Mat or towel (or whatever is available for a little cushioning from the floor)

Description

- Lie on the floor on your right side and place your right hand on your left side at your waist.
- Place your left hand on the floor in front of your right shoulder.
- Keeps your legs slightly bent and make sure the pelvis is stacked with the left hip bone aligned over the right hip bone (a).
- Inhale to prepare.
- Exhale to engage as you press into your left hand and straighten your left arm to push your body up and off the floor (b).

Safety Considerations

If you feel any pressure in your pelvis, limit your range of motion or do the other triceps exercises instead.

Increase Difficulty

Extend the legs straight out.

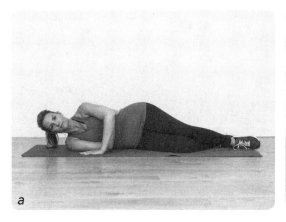
a

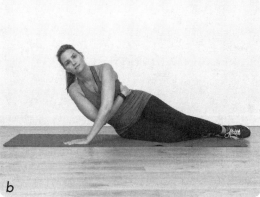
b

Skull Crusher on Stability Ball With Hip Thrust

Focus and Benefits

Combining two exercises in one is efficient and increases the challenge by incorporating the whole body, not just working the arms.

Equipment

Stability ball and dumbbells

Description

- Place a stability ball on the floor. Then place a dumbbell on the floor on either side of you within your reach and squat with your back facing the stability ball.
- Grab the dumbbells and hold them close into you as you lean back so your upper back and head are supported by the ball.
- Lift your bum and walk your feet out until your torso is parallel to the floor and your head and back of your shoulders are on top of the ball.
- Extend and straighten both arms toward the ceiling (a).
- Inhale to expand as you bend the elbows to lower the weights toward your ears, keeping your arms parallel to each other. At the same time, drop your bum slightly toward the floor (b).
- Exhale to engage as you thrust your hips up and simultaneously straighten both arms.

Safety Considerations

- If you feel unstable, you can wedge the ball in a corner or place it against a wall.
- You can also do this with a regular bench for added stability.

Increase Difficulty

- Increase the weight of the dumbbells.
- Increase the number of reps.

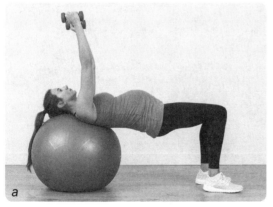
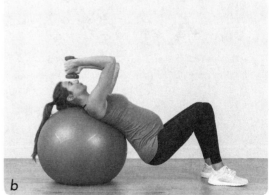

a

b

Crab Walk

Focus and Benefits

This exercise is like a reverse plank and is a good full-body challenge with a little extra work targeted to the triceps and shoulders.

Equipment

None

Description

- Sit on the floor with your knees bent and your arms behind you with your fingers pointing toward your feet.
- Inhale to prepare.
- Exhale to engage and lift your bum off the floor so you are supporting yourself just on your hands and feet.
- Walk 10 steps forward and 10 steps backward.

Safety Considerations

Omit this exercise if you feel too much strain on your shoulders.

Increase Difficulty

Take five more steps each direction.

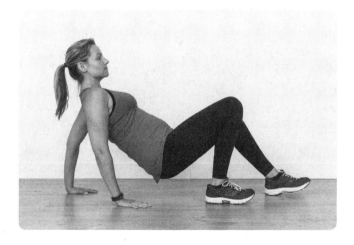

Triceps Press on BOSU

Focus and Benefits

The addition of the BOSU adds an element of instability to help challenge your whole body while still targeting the triceps.

Equipment

BOSU and dumbbells

Description

- Place a BOSU on the floor and sit on your side in front of it.
- Place your dumbbells on the floor next to you.
- Lower your head to the BOSU then roll over so the back of your head is on the BOSU. Grab a dumbbell in each hand, then press your hips up toward the ceiling so you are in a tabletop position.
- Inhale to prepare as you bend the elbows and lower the dumbbells toward your chest (a).
- Exhale to engage as you press the dumbbells back up toward the ceiling. You will keep your hips off the floor the entire time and only move your elbows (b).

Safety Considerations

- You can lower your hips down and keep your bum on the floor if you need a break.
- Ensure that you have a secure grip on the dumbbells.

Increase Difficulty

- Increase the number of reps.
- Grab a heavier set of dumbbells.

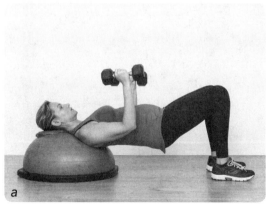
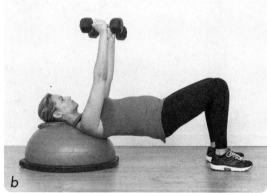

a b

Stationary Lunge With Overhead Triceps Extension

Focus and Benefits

Target the legs, glutes, and triceps all at once with this great exercise.

Equipment

Dumbbell

Description

- Hold one dumbbell with both hands at either end.
- Extend and straighten both arms to lift the weight over your head. Your elbows will be pointing forward when the weight is raised and arms are parallel.
- Stand in a neutral posture and extend one leg behind you with the heel up *(a)*.
- Inhale to expand as you bend the back leg to lower into a lunge. Simultaneously bend both elbows to lower the weight behind your head *(b)*.
- Exhale to engage as you straighten the arms to raise the weight and at the same time straighten your front leg to press up from the lunge.

Safety Considerations

- If you find it challenging to straighten your arms without arching your back then stick to either a stationary lunge or a standing triceps extension.
- If you feel unstable you can narrow the stance or stick to a standing triceps extension.

Increase Difficulty

- Place your front foot on a BOSU for an added challenge.
- Increase the weight.
- Increase the number of reps.

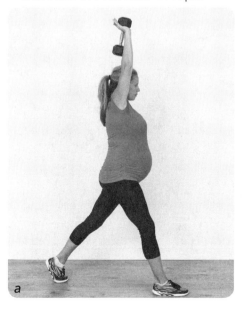
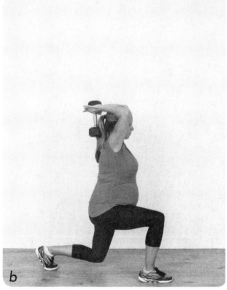

SHOULDERS

Most people, pregnant or not, have rounded shoulders and could do with some stretching for the chest and front of the shoulders as well as some strengthening of the middle and back parts of the shoulders. Your shoulders will be working a lot with all the lifting and carrying you will be doing, so you want them strong and supple!

Standing Upright Row With Band

Focus and Benefits

This exercise really targets the middle and back of the shoulders and will help with all the lifting you will be doing!

Equipment

Resistance band

Description

- Stand tall with a neutral pelvis and your feet pelvis-width apart.
- Step on the middle of the resistance band and grab one end of the band in each hand with your palms facing behind you (a).
- Inhale to prepare.
- Exhale to engage and then pull up on the band, leading with your elbows to bring your hands up to chest height (b).

Safety Considerations

- If you have any pain in the shoulders, avoid this exercise.
- Keep your shoulders away from your ears and neck relaxed.

Increase Difficulty

- Choose a thicker resistance band for greater resistance.
- Increase the number of reps.

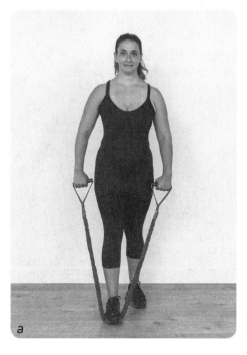
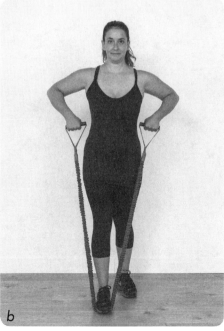

a

b

Lateral Raise

Focus and Benefits

This is another great exercise for the middle of the shoulders to improve strength, endurance, and definition.

Equipment

Dumbbells

Description

- Stand tall with feet pelvis-width apart and a neutral pelvis.
- Hold a dumbbell in each hand with your arms at your sides and palms facing your body (a).
- Inhale to prepare.
- Exhale to engage then lift your arms to the sides away from your body to bring your hands to shoulder height, making the letter "T" with your arms and body (b).

Safety Considerations

- If you have any pain in the shoulders avoid this exercise.
- Keep your shoulders away from your ears and neck relaxed.

Increase Difficulty

- Choose heavier weights for greater resistance.
- Increase the number of reps.
- Try raising the weights while standing on one leg.

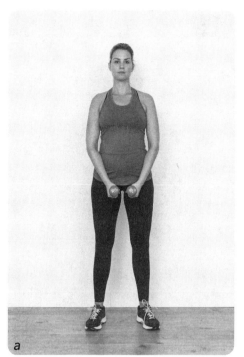
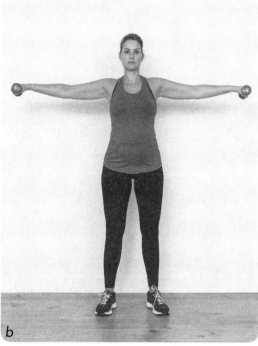

a

b

Here is a fantastic core, leg, and shoulder exercise that will really challenge you! Grab a light dumbbell—maybe five pounds (2 kg)—in both hands and extend your arms straight out in front of you at shoulder height. Inhale to expand as you squat down. Hold the squat but not your breath. Now, while keeping the arms straight, circle the weight in one direction for 10 reps then switch and circle them in the other direction for 10 reps. Stand back up and take a break. Tough isn't it? We don't have you breathing with the core breath here—just breathe and know that your pelvic floor is working. If you feel any heaviness in your pelvic floor you can do this with a smaller squat or just standing with feet pelvis-width apart.

Seated Shoulder Press

Focus and Benefits

While the focus is on the middle shoulder, this exercise really works the entire shoulder area.

Equipment

Dumbbells and a stability ball or a chair

Description

- Sit on a stability ball or a chair with a neutral pelvis.
- With your arms at your sides, hold a dumbbell in each hand and bend your elbows to raise the dumbbells to about shoulder height with the palms facing forward (a).
- Inhale to prepare.
- Exhale to engage and extend and straighten the arms to press the dumbbells up toward the ceiling (b).

Safety Considerations

Ensure you do not arch your back as you lift.

Increase Difficulty

- Choose heavier dumbbells for more challenge.
- Increase the number of reps.
- Try standing.

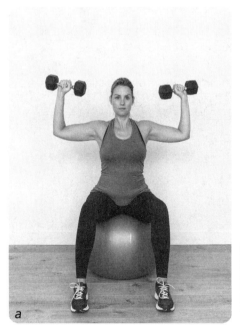

a

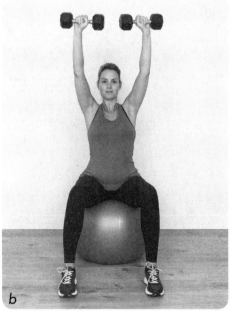

b

Alternating Front Raise

Focus and Benefits

The front part of the shoulder is targeted in this exercise, which helps get you ready for lifting.

Equipment

Dumbbells

Description

- Stand tall with feet pelvis-width apart and with the pelvis in a neutral position.
- Hold a dumbbell in each hand with palms resting on the front of your thighs (a).
- Inhale to prepare.
- Exhale to engage then lift your right arm straight out in front of you to raise the weight to shoulder height (b).
- Inhale and return the arm to the start.
- Repeat on the other side.

Safety Considerations

- If you have any pain in the shoulders avoid this exercise.
- Ensure you do not sway or arch your back.
- You can choose to do this exercise seated on a chair or stability ball if you feel unstable or you are arching your back.

Increase Difficulty

- Choose heavier weights for greater resistance.
- Increase the number of reps.
- Try standing on one leg while performing the raise.
- Lift both arms at the same time.

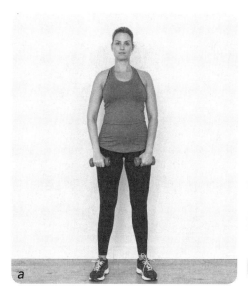
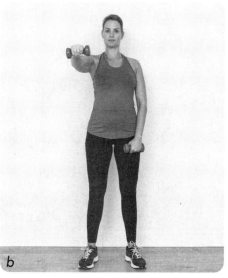

a

b

Bent-Arm Lateral Raise

Focus and Benefits

Instead of the straight-arm raise described in the previous exercise, this exercise is a different way to target the middle shoulder muscles. The shorter lever length you get by bending your arms means you can often lift a bit heavier weight.

Equipment

Dumbbells

Description

- Stand with feet pelvis-width apart and a neutral pelvis.
- Hold a dumbbell in each hand with your arms at your sides and bent at 90 degrees with your palms facing each other *(a)*.
- Inhale to prepare.
- Exhale to engage and lift the elbows to shoulder height while maintaining the 90-degree angle *(b)*.
- Form the letter "T" as in the regular lateral raise.

Safety Considerations

- If you have any pain in the shoulders avoid this exercise.
- You can choose to do this exercise seated on a chair or stability ball if needed.

Increase Difficulty

- Choose heavier weights for greater resistance.
- Increase the number of reps.

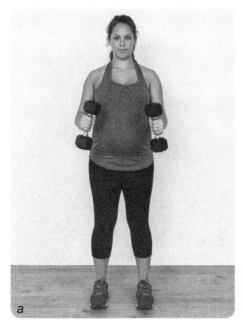
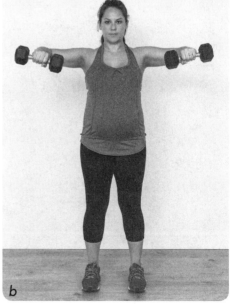

Rear Crescent Lunge

Focus and Benefits

This is a great way to stretch the front body—the abdomen, front of the pelvis and chest.

Equipment

None

Description

- Stand with your feet pelvis-width apart.
- Extend your right leg back behind you in a lunge position while you simultaneously reach both arms up overhead, keeping the arms straight.
- Hold for three to five seconds, then return to the starting position and repeat on the other side.

Safety Considerations

Narrow the stance if you feel unsteady.

Increase Difficulty

- Hold the pose longer.

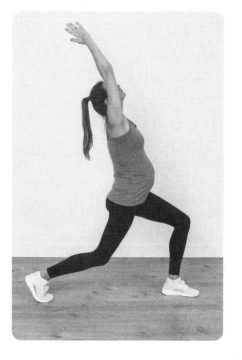

CHALLENGE YOURSELF As a busy mom, you will often find yourself in odd positions while you try to hold a sleeping baby and reach for a glass on the top shelf or maybe slide something out of the way with your foot and distract your child with your hands. Here is a great exercise that will work your whole body but also does a good job at working those shoulders, readying them for reaching. Place a gliding disc or a small hand towel on the floor and put your left toes on it. Transfer your weight to your right leg. Inhale to expand as you reach your left leg behind you by gliding your foot back while also reaching both arms out in front of you. Exhale to engage as you lower the arms and draw the left foot forward to the starting position. You get some nice length in the front of your body as you inhale and some gentle contraction of the core as you exhale. Do 10 to 12 reps on each side.

8

Strength and Endurance for the Lower Body

Many of the physical changes in pregnancy occur in the lower body, namely the feet and the pelvis. The ever-increasing load that the body must adapt to can create compensations that contribute to many of the aches and pains women think are normal in pregnancy and motherhood. The postural changes, the hormonal changes, the increased weight, and the shifting center of gravity all place additional challenges on the lower body, such as sacroiliac joint pain, hip pain, lower- back pain, and symphysis pubis dysfunction (pain in the pubic joint).

Your feet carry you from point A to point B each and every day, so they deserve some TLC beyond the occasional pedicure. Your feet have most likely been cooped up in shoes for most of your life and as a result, the muscles in your feet that should be working to support you are most likely deconditioned due to the "casting" (like a cast for a broken bone) effect that shoes create. Ideally, shoes should have a thin, flexible sole and a wide toe box that allow for movement and use of the foot. Standard footwear is often rigid and supportive, with a narrow toe box that essentially holds your foot in a given position, not allowing the muscles to do their job. There are 19 muscles and 26 bones in each foot. Ideally, the feet have freedom to respond to the ever-changing ground beneath us and ensure we don't fall. When our feet are held in a fixed position in a shoe, the muscles do not move using their full range of motion; therefore, compensations can develop and the foot essentially becomes deconditioned. When the shifting center of gravity is added to the deconditioned foot, your feet will probably start to protest with aches and pains! Transitioning to minimal shoes and spending more time "barefoot and pregnant" can help build the muscles in the feet. Using small balls to roll under the feet can help relieve the tension that develops in pregnancy and it feels fantastic! Happy healthy feet that have freedom of movement contribute to optimal posture, which in turn allows the muscles in the legs and the core to work as they should.

The legs have some of the largest muscles in the body, and you want these muscles to be strong and have endurance for labor. Remaining active in birth is essential and having legs that can hold you in different positions such as squatting, kneeling, or staggered standing will make for an overall easier labor. Often women view birth as something done lying down, when really it should be seen as a dynamic process. It is called labor for a reason. By building strength and muscular endurance in your legs during pregnancy, you will be prepared for the physical demands of birth, you will feel better in your pregnancy, and you will recover more quickly postpartum.

The best way to train the legs is to walk every day and choose exercises that mimic the various birth positions you may use in labor. Remember the principle of specificity? Use the body how it will be used in the event you are training for. In birth, you will be walking, squatting, holding staggered-stance positions, spending time kneeling or supported on all fours, and maybe even lying on your side. Make sure that your exercise choices in pregnancy prepare you for this. The lower body really takes on the bulk of the workload in labor, so it is essential to focus a lot of your training on the lower half of the body. Strength, length, and endurance are all key, so include progressions in the number of reps and the length of time to hold certain positions as well as increasing the amount of stretching and release work to keep the muscles supple and tension free.

Let's take a look at the exercises you can use to get your lower body ready for labor and motherhood. Also, remember to add in the core breath—inhale to expand then exhale to engage just before you exert the force (see chapter 6 for more about core breath). You can turn almost any exercise into a core and pelvic floor exercise by adding in the core breath!

Calf Raise With Stability Ball

Focus and Benefits

- Builds strength and endurance in the calves and encourages blood circulation to help minimize varicose veins.
- Challenges your balance

Equipment

Stability ball

Description

- Place a stability ball between your chest and a wall with your forearms placed on the front of the ball and arms at 90 degrees.
- Step back about one foot so that your body is slightly angled into the ball. Stand tall with your feet pelvis-width apart and pointed forward (a).
- Inhale to expand and prepare.
- Exhale to engage as you press up onto your toes (either both feet or just one at a time), keeping your legs straight (b).

Safety Considerations

Start with your feet close enough to the wall so you keep a 90-degree angle in your ankles. You can step back farther, increasing the lean and decreasing the angle in your ankles, as you progress.

Increase Difficulty

- Step back from the wall a little farther.
- Do one leg at a time to really challenge your balance and core.

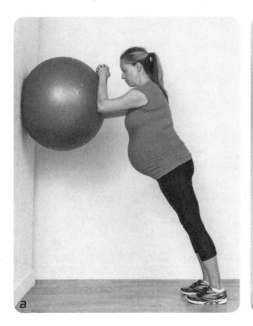
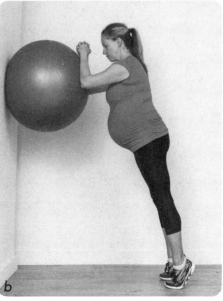

Stability Ball Squat

Focus and Benefits

- Builds strength and endurance in the quads, hamstrings, and glutes
- Trains your body for functional movements
- Prepares you for squatting in labor

Equipment

Stability ball

Description

- Stand near a wall with your back facing the wall. Hold a stability ball against your lower back, with the bottom of your shoulder blades touching the ball. Back up until you contact the wall. Stand tall with your feet pelvis-width apart and pointing forward (a).
- Inhale to expand as you bend your knees and lower down, pressing your bum back and keeping your weight in your heels (b).
- Exhale to engage as you straighten your legs to press back up.
- You may also work at holding a static squat position, where you lower down and then hold the squat for 10 to 30 seconds.

Safety Considerations

Start with your feet far enough in front of you so your knees move forward, or track, only as far as your mid-foot. You want to avoid having your knees remain over your ankles. Tracking too far forward also places the bulk of the work in the quads, when it should really be the glutes and hamstrings that do the majority of the work.

Increase Difficulty

- Try squats without the ball.
- Try squatting on a BOSU with the dome up for an even greater challenge. You may want to take a wider stance where the feet are placed more toward the sides of the ball. Ensure, as above, that your knees do not move forward past your toes. Note that this is not to be done in the second or third trimester; the added instability can increase the risk of falling.

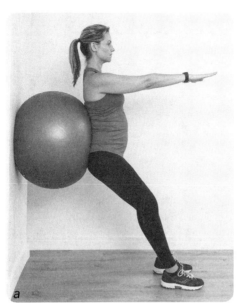

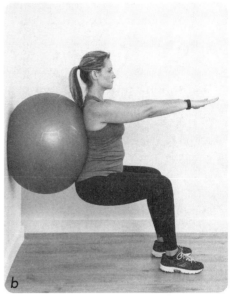

CHALLENGE YOURSELF Body-weight squats are challenging, and the fact that your body weight is increasing throughout your pregnancy means you are naturally progressing to increased loads without even doing anything different! You can up the ante even more by adding dumbbells in your hands. Try one in each hand to start. From there you can progress to holding a dumbbell in one hand only to start training you for the many uneven loads you will face in motherhood.

Stability Ball Lunge

Focus and Benefits

- Builds strength and muscular endurance in quads, hamstrings, and glutes
- Trains the body for functional movements
- Prepares you for asymmetric standing birth positions

Equipment

Stability ball

Description

- Stand near a wall with your back facing the wall. Hold a stability ball against your lower back, with the bottom of your shoulder blades touching the ball. Back up until you contact the wall. Stand tall and do not lean forward.
- Place your right foot forward and your left foot behind you with the toes of your left foot on the floor and the heel up so you are in a split stance (a).
- Inhale to expand as you bend your right leg to lower down, pressing your bum back and keeping the weight in your right heel. The right knee moves forward or tracks over your ankle rather than your toes in the deepest part of the lunge to protect your knees and ensure the load is distributed more in the glutes and hamstrings than in the quads (b).
- Exhale to engage as you straighten your right leg to press back up.

Safety Considerations

Ensure your beginning stance is wide enough to allow for proper tracking of the front knee. The front knee should move on an imaginary line between your first and second toes but should not move forward beyond the toes.

Increase Difficulty

- Try a stationary lunge with no ball.
- Use dumbbells in both hands or in just one hand to help your body train for uneven loads, such as carrying a car seat.

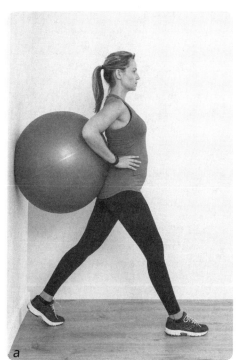 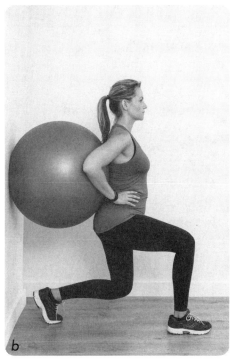

Standing Hamstring Curl With Stability Ball

Focus and Benefits

- Builds strength and endurance in the hamstrings
- Builds strength and endurance in the lateral hip muscles of the standing leg
- Helps with core strength

Equipment

Stability ball

Description

- Stand with your back against a wall and place the stability ball on the floor in front of you within reach of one of your feet. Place that foot on top of the ball and stabilize your weight over your standing leg. Use your working leg to roll the ball close enough so your working knee is bent at 90 degrees.
- Inhale to prepare as you roll the ball away from you *(a)*.
- Exhale, dig your heel into the ball, and roll the ball back in until your working knee is at 90 degrees *(b)*.

Safety Considerations

If you are having balance issues, place one hand on a chair for stability.

Increase Difficulty

- Do a biceps curl with a dumbbell in one or both hands at the same time.
- Stand away from the wall with your right side toward the wall and your right hand on the wall for support.
- Stand away from the wall with no hands on the wall to really challenge your core stability and balance.

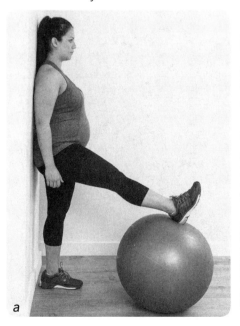
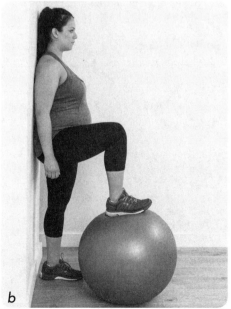

a

b

Donkey Kick

Focus and Benefits

- Builds strength and endurance in the hamstrings
- Builds strength in the glutes.
- Challenges the core and low back

Equipment

Mat

Description

- Kneel on the floor in an upright position.
- Perform a core breath to create tension across your lower abdominals.
- While you maintain the tension, lower your hands to the floor, and walk out to all fours so that your hands are under your shoulders and your knees are under your hips *(a)*.
- Inhale to prepare.
- Exhale and bend and lift one knee to bring the sole of the foot toward the ceiling *(b)*.
- Inhale to expand as you lower the knee back down.

Safety Considerations

This exercise is not recommended after the first trimester. While it is perfectly safe, it does place an additional load on the linea alba in the abdomen, which may increase the stretch. This could potentially increase the distance between the two rectus muscles. We recommend doing a standing hip extension exercise as an alternative.

Increase Difficulty

- Try kneeling on the dome of a BOSU.
- Try keeping a straight leg. This increases the lever length, which can make it more challenging. You may also wish to add an ankle weight for increased resistance.

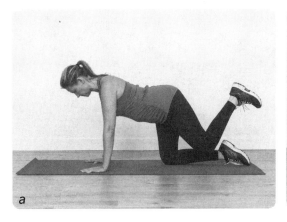
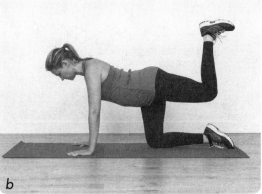

a b

Standing Hip Abduction With Ball

Focus and Benefits
- Builds strength and endurance for glutes and abductors
- Helps maintain the ability to transfer load from one leg to the other

Equipment
Stability ball

Description
- Stand with your right side facing a wall and with the feet together. Place one hand on the wall for support. Do not lean into the wall.
- Place a stability ball against the wall just above the right knee.
- Bend your right knee 90 degrees and keep your thighs parallel *(a)*.
- Keep your hips square and facing forward.
- Inhale to prepare.
- Exhale and press the ball against the wall with the bent right leg *(b)*.

Safety Considerations
Maintain proper posture throughout so you don't strain your back.

Increase Difficulty
- Wrap a resistance band around your knees or ankles to increase the intensity.
- Stand on the dome of a BOSU to challenge your balance and stability (not recommended in the second and third trimesters).

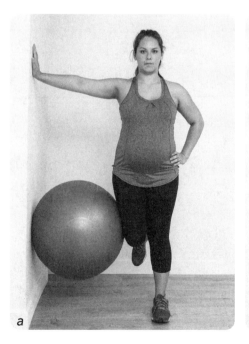
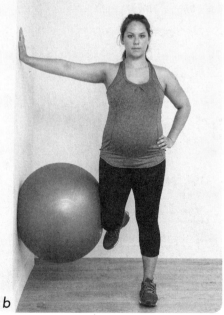

a

b

Seated Hip Abduction

Focus and Benefits
- Builds strength and endurance in the lateral hip muscles
- Develops the glutes and pelvic floor
- Prepares you for labor positions

Equipment
Chair or stability ball and a resistance band

Description
- Sit with a neutral pelvis on a chair or a stability ball with your feet pelvis-width apart.
- Place a resistance band around your thighs so that it rests just above your knees (a).
- Inhale to expand and prepare.
- Exhale to engage and then press your thighs outward against the band (b).
- Inhale to expand as you allow the thighs to return to center.

Safety Considerations
- If you are feeling unsteady, use a chair instead of a stability ball.
- You can also wedge the ball into a corner for more stability.
- Holding the ball with your hands may help you feel more steady.

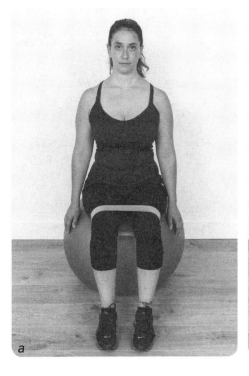

a

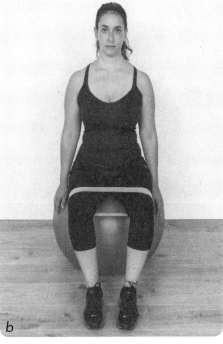

b

Seated Hip Adduction

Focus and Benefits
- Builds and strengthens the adductors
- Recruits the pelvic floor

Equipment
Stability ball and a smaller ball such as a soccer ball, bender ball, or Pilates ball

Description
- Sit tall on a stability ball with your pelvis untucked and place your feet comfortably on the floor about one foot apart. Place your hands on both sides of the ball.
- Place a small ball between your knees (a).
- Inhale to prepare.
- Exhale and squeeze the ball between your knees (b).

Safety Considerations
Place the stability ball against a wall for more stability. If this brings on pelvic pain, discontinue this exercise.

Increase Difficulty
- Don't hold the stability ball.
- Try this exercise in a standing position with a small ball between the legs.

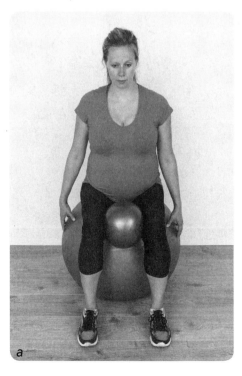
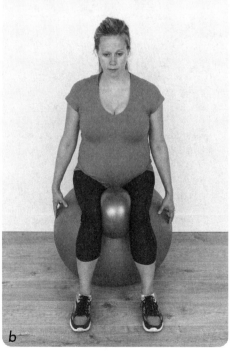

Walking Lunge

Focus and Benefits
- Builds strength and endurance in the legs
- Develops your glutes and pelvic floor
- Trains your balance and builds pelvic stability

Description
- Stand with your feet pelvis-width apart and your arms on your hips or hanging down at your sides.
- Inhale to prepare.
- Exhale as you step forward, then inhale and bend your knees to lower down, pressing your bum back and keeping your weight in your front heel. The front knee stays aligned over the ankle rather than moving over the toes in the deepest part of the lunge to protect the knee and ensure the load is distributed more in the glutes and hamstrings than in the quads (a).
- Exhale to engage and slightly straighten your legs to begin moving forward. Press up with and then lift your back leg so it can move forward and transition from being the back leg to being the front leg (b).

Safety Considerations
If you feel unstable stay with the stationary lunge or perform these next to a wall that you can reach out to for balance if needed.

Increase Difficulty
- Use dumbbells in both hands or in just one hand to help your body train for uneven loads, such as carrying a car seat.
- Hold a bolster in your arms to mimic a baby. This not only adds resistance but also trains you for the way you will move in motherhood.

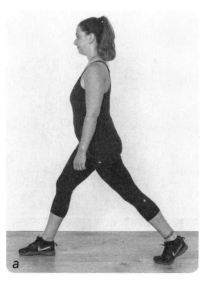
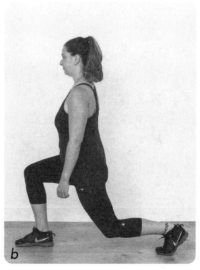

a

b

Deadlift

Focus and Benefits

- Builds strength and endurance in the glutes, and lower back
- Prepares you for getting your baby into and out of the crib or bassinette

Equipment

Barbell

Description

- Stand with your feet pelvis-width apart and your legs straight.
- Hold a barbell and let it rest on the front of your thighs *(a)*.
- Inhale to expand as you hinge forward from the hips and slide the barbell along the front of your legs toward the floor while keeping the pelvis neutral.
- Allow your pelvis to move backward while keeping your knees straight (but not locked).
- Keep your body weight in front of you and reach gradually lower and more forward until you feel a nice stretch in the back of the hamstrings *(b)*.
- Exhale to engage and use your glutes to bring you back to upright.

Safety Considerations

Ensure your pelvis stays in a neutral position and your shoulders stay back.

Increase Difficulty

- Increase the weight you are lifting.
- Use a bolster and place it in a crib to mimic your baby. This adds resistance but also trains you for the movement you will do many times in motherhood.

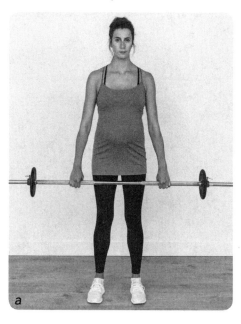
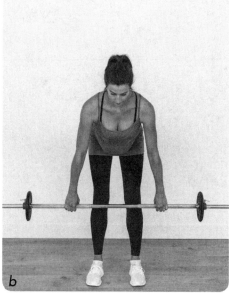

a

b

Straight-Leg Bridge With Stability Ball

Focus and Benefits

- Builds strength and endurance in the hamstrings
- Works your lower body and core together

Equipment

Stability ball and a mat

Description

- Lie on your back and place the back of your calves on top of the ball. Your arms are at your sides with the palms down on the floor (a).
- Inhale to prepare.
- Exhale to engage and press the hips up toward the ceiling (b).
- Inhale to expand and allow the hips to return to the starting position with control.

Safety Considerations

If you are feeling unsteady, do this exercise with the ball wedged into a corner.

Increase Difficulty

- Once you lift your bum off the floor you can then lift one leg off the ball while keeping the ball stable.
- Keep both legs on the ball then curl your heels into your bum for a hamstring curl.

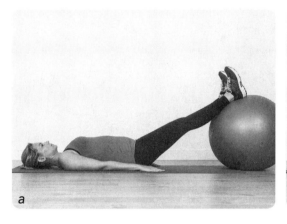
a

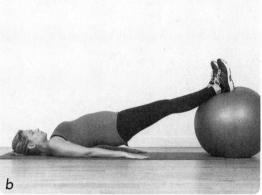
b

Deadlift and Back Row

Focus and Benefits

- Builds strength and endurance in the glutes, low back and upper back
- Prepares you for getting your baby into and out of the crib or bassinette

Equipment

Two dumbbells

Description

- Stand with feet pelvis-width apart and hold a dumbbell in each hand resting on the front of your thighs *(a)*.
- Inhale to expand as you hinge forward from the hips while keeping a neutral pelvis and begin to lower the dumbbells.
- Keep the dumbbells close to your legs (imagine shaving your legs).
- Allow your pelvis to move backward while keeping your knees straight (but not locked). Keep your body weight in front of you and the dumbbells toward the floor *(b)*.
- In the hinged position, exhale to engage and perform a back row with the dumbbells, driving the elbows back and squeezing your shoulder blades *(c)*.
- Inhale and extend the dumbbells back toward the floor.
- Exhale to engage and use your glutes to bring you back to upright.

Safety Considerations

Ensure the pelvis stays in a neutral position and your shoulders stay back while you are in the hinged position.

Increase Difficulty

- Perform this exercise on a BOSU with the dome up.
- You can perform a single-leg deadlift as well (but not on a BOSU).

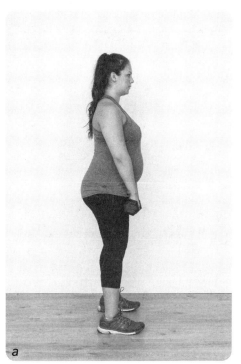

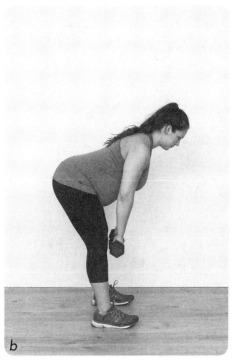

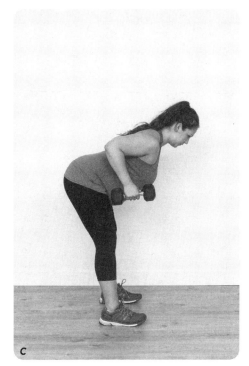

Frankenstein Walk

Focus and Benefits

- Builds strength and endurance in the lateral hips
- Improves your walking mechanics
- Challenges the core

Equipment

Resistance band

Description

- Place a resistance band around your thighs just above your knees with enough tension to hold it there while keeping your feet pelvis-width apart and your hands on your hips (a).
- Step to the right with your right leg, keeping your leg straight and stretching the band further (b).
- Land on the outside edge of your right foot, then lift your left leg and bring it in toward the midline, but not so close to your right leg that the resistance band slips down.
- Take four steps in one direction then step toward the opposite direction, breathing as you need to.
- Do five cycles of four steps per side.

Safety Considerations

Avoid this exercise if you have pain in your pubic joint. Adjust the band around the thighs if pain in knees occurs

Increase Difficulty

- Increase the resistance of your band.
- Add a squat in between each step.
- Increase the number of steps in each direction.

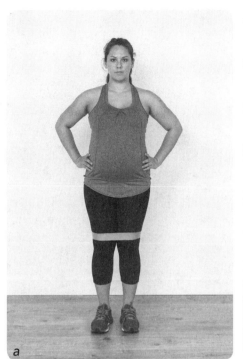 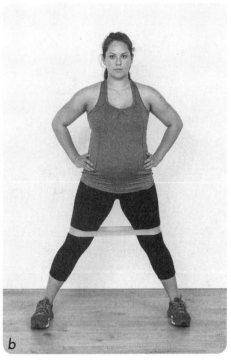

Squat on BOSU

Focus and Benefits

- Builds strength and endurance in the legs and core
- Challenges your balance

Equipment

BOSU

Description

- Place the BOSU on the floor with the dome up.
- First, place one foot on the BOSU and then place the other. Once stabilized, your feet should be pelvis-width apart and your arms should be out in front (a).
- Inhale as you sit your bum back and lower down into a squat, ensuring your knees do not move forward beyond your toes (b).
- Exhale to engage and straighten your legs to press back up to standing.

Safety Considerations

- Place the BOSU close to a wall so you can have one hand on the wall for balance if needed.
- This exercise is not recommended in the second and third trimesters.

Increase Difficulty

- Use dumbbells in both hands or in just one hand to help your body train for uneven loads, such as carrying a car seat.
- Hold the lowest part of the squat for three to five seconds before standing up.

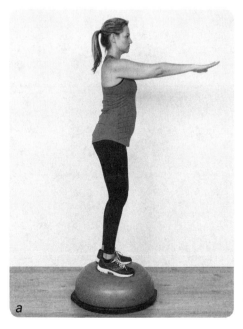
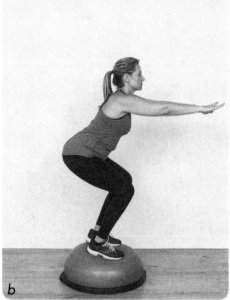

a

b

Stationary Lunge With One Foot on BOSU

Focus and Benefits

- Builds strength and endurance in the lower body
- Challenges the core
- Trains your balance

Equipment

BOSU

Description

- Place a BOSU on the ground with the dome up.
- Place your right foot on the top of the BOSU so your anklebone is lined up with the center circle.
- Take a long step back with your left leg so only the toes of the left foot are on the ground (the left heel is raised) (a).
- Inhale as you lead with the back leg and bend your knees to lower down into a lunge (b).
- Exhale to engage as you press with the front leg and straighten up to the starting position.
- Repeat on the other leg.

Safety Considerations

Place the BOSU close to a wall so you can use the wall for support. This is safe for all trimesters as you have one foot on the ground at all times.

Increase Difficulty

- Use dumbbells in both hands or in just one hand to help your body train for uneven loads, such as carrying a car seat.
- Try the exercise with the BOSU dome down for added instability and challenge.

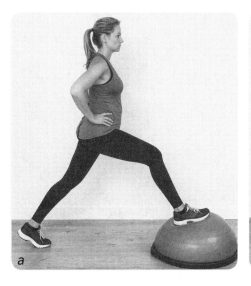
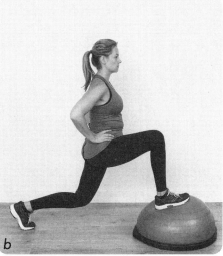

a

b

Deadlift on BOSU

Focus and Benefits

- Builds strength and endurance in the glutes
- Challenges the core
- Actively stretches the hamstrings

Equipment

BOSU and dumbbells

Description

- Place a BOSU on the ground with the dome up.
- Stand on top of the BOSU with the feet pelvis-width apart and hold a dumbbell in each hand, resting the palms on the front of your thighs *(a)*.
- Inhale as you hinge at the hips, keeping the legs straight (but not locked).
- Slide the dumbbells along the front of your legs (think shaving your legs) until you get a nice stretch in the back of your hamstrings *(b)*.
- Exhale to engage and use the glutes as you return to the starting position.

Safety Considerations

Place the BOSU close to a wall so you can use the wall for support. Note that this exercise is not recommended in the second and third trimesters.

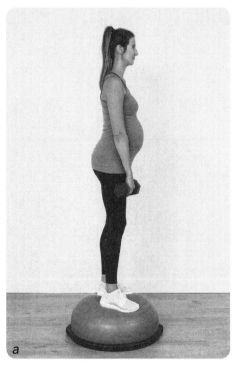
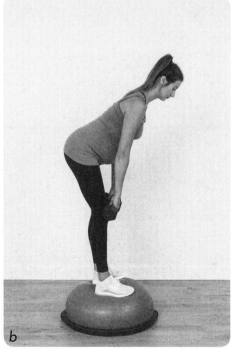

Hip Thrust

Focus and Benefits
- Builds strength and endurance in the glutes
- Challenges the core

Equipment
Stability Ball

Description
- Place the stability ball on the floor.
- Sit on the floor in front of the ball, then rest your head on the ball and lift your bum off the floor a few inches (a).
- Inhale to prepare.
- Exhale to engage and thrust your hips up toward the ceiling (b).
- Inhale to expand as you lower your hips back down, stopping just before they reach the floor.

Safety Considerations
You can do this exercise on a bench if you feel unstable with the ball.

Increase Difficulty
In the first and second trimester, you may wish to add a weighted sandbag on your hips for added resistance.

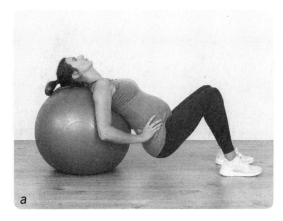
a

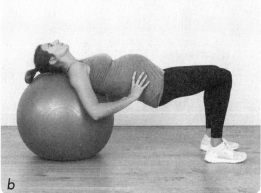
b

One-Leg Deadlift

Focus and Benefits

- Builds strength and endurance in the legs and glutes
- Challenges the core and balance

Equipment

Dumbbell

Description

- Stand with feet pelvis-width apart and the pelvis in a neutral position.
- Place a dumbbell on its end on the floor in front of you (a).
- Inhale to expand as you tip forward allowing your right leg to float toward the ceiling and keeping your left hip aligned with the right.
- Extend your right arm to reach and tap the end of the dumbbell as you lower down (b).
- Exhale to engage and push through the left leg as you return to the standing position.
- Do 10 reps and then repeat on other leg.

Safety Considerations

Ensure the hips remain square and do not allow the pelvis to rotate.

Increase Difficulty

Instead of leaving the dumbbell on the floor, hold it in both hands, or use two dumbbells and hold one in each hand.

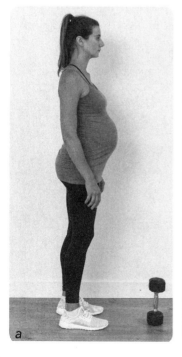

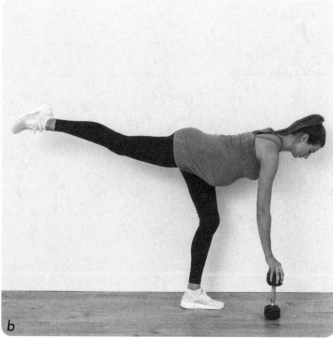

Kneeling Hover

Focus and Benefits
- Builds strength and endurance in the legs and glutes
- Prepares you for kneeling and all-fours labor positions

Equipment
Mat

Description
- Kneel on your mat with your feet together and knees slightly wider than hip-width apart. Allow your bum to rest on your feet.
- Place your hands on your hips *(a)*.
- Inhale to expand to prepare.
- Exhale to engage and lift your bum away from your feet to come in to a tall kneeling position *(b)*.
- Inhale to expand and lower back down to the starting position.

Safety Considerations
If you have any pain in the pubic joint, narrow the distance between the knees or simply avoid this exercise. You can also place a pillow between your bum and your feet if you feel too much pressure in your knees while sitting on your feet.

Increase Difficulty
Perform the movement slower and more controlled both up and down.

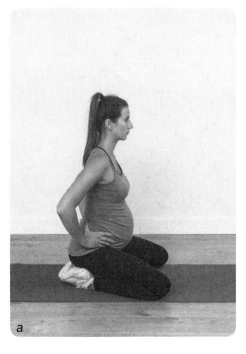

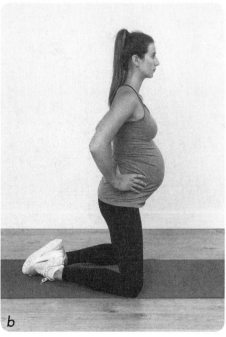

Monster Walk

Focus and Benefits
- Builds strength and endurance in the legs, and glutes
- Gets you ready for holding squat and kneeling positions in labor
- Challenges the core

Equipment
Resistance band

Description
- Place a resistance band around your thighs just above your knees.
- Bend knees so you are in a semi-squat position *(a)*.
- Staying in the semi-squat, walk by taking small steps forward one leg at a time while keeping tension in the band *(b)*.
- Take five steps with each leg then walk backwards to the start, keeping tension in the band.

Safety Considerations
Ensure the band is above the knees. Avoid this exercise if it produces pubic joint pain.

Increase Difficulty
- Use a greater resistance exercise band.
- Increase the number of steps.

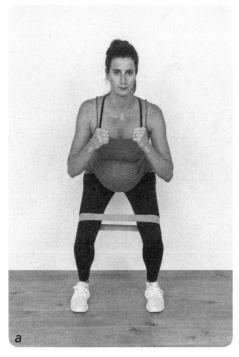
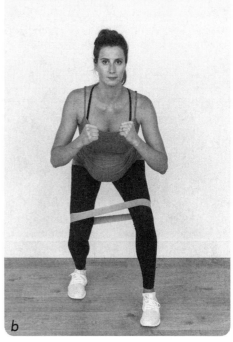

a

b

Functional Movement for Motherhood

9

Training is important because it is the key to being prepared for any new sport, competition, or activity. The more often you perform a task in a certain sequence, the better you will perform that task. We have talked about training for labor and birth throughout this book, and now there is one more component you need to train for: motherhood. As a new mom, you will face many new physical challenges—lifting the car seat, carrying the baby and a diaper bag, pushing and pulling the stroller, twisting to put the soother back in your baby's mouth, getting up off the floor, etc.— and you'll start doing these on an exhausted body that has just undergone arguably the most challenging event there is! The good news is muscles have memory, and training them in these movement sequences before the big day will help ensure that your recovery goes smoothly and your body remembers how to engage optimally for the task at hand.

After the birth of your baby, regardless of whether it was a vaginal or a cesarean birth, the Core 4 muscles will be stretched, some tissues may be cut, and your muscles will not be working as well as they normally do. Well-trained muscles heal more efficiently than untrained muscles, so trust that your preparation in pregnancy will support your recovery and your transition into motherhood.

The first thing you need to do is make sure you are doing the core breath exercise daily and incorporating it into movement. This creates synergy between the deepest layer of your core system, bringing together your diaphragm, pelvic floor, deep abdominals, and multifidus. If you haven't started doing it yet, go back to chapter 6 where we introduced you to your core breath.

Next, the movements of motherhood are broken down into exercises you perform to increase your strength, endurance, and flexibility. Functional movements are built gradually so you will be able to execute the full movements once your baby is born. We recommend that you begin each workout session with some release work (see chapter 5), because muscles that are too tight do not perform well. By releasing any tension first, the muscles have the freedom to work as they should.

After the release work you can move on to the exercises that prepare you for the movements you will do in motherhood. A key component here is to make sure you can accomplish each exercise with perfect form. It is absolutely useless and downright harmful if you continue an exercise with bad form. You are just teaching your body to compensate. If your form is compromised, decrease the load or amount of weight, or the number of reps and do only as much as you can do perfectly. And remember, you are pregnant. This means that even though you could do your usual routine yesterday, today is a whole new day with a whole new body. Embrace the changes and challenges, respect your limitations, and gently nudge your boundaries each day.

In the previous chapters, you learned exercises for upper- and lower-body strengthening. We are going to refer back to those for the prerequisite movements or exercises as we break down the movements for motherhood. The general components to the movements for motherhood are listed below, followed by the specific exercises that will prepare you for the functional movements of motherhood.

- *Squat*—bending at the hips and knees to lower yourself down toward the floor
- *Lift*—picking something up and bringing it into your arms
- *Carry*—holding something in your arms
- *Push*—moving something away from your body
- *Pull*—bringing something closer to your body
- *Rotate*—turning your upper body to the left or right while keeping your lower body relatively stationary
- *Bend*—rounding out the spine (forward) or extending through the spine (backward)
- *Pick up*—grasping something or someone off the ground or other lower surface
- *Balance*—maintaining an upright position despite the lack of physical support or in the face of a base-of-support perturbation (something pushing or pulling you off balance)

Baby and Bag Carry

When carrying baby and a diaper bag, the typical pattern is to jut out one hip and hook baby on it, and then sling the diaper bag over the opposite shoulder. Occasionally, both are carried on the same side. However, ideally you would carry your baby in front centered over your body in a carrier or in your arms and the diaper bag in back as a backpack. This distributes the weight a little more evenly and allows for more symmetrical movement. Be careful to follow the instructions on baby carriers and use as directed.

Prerequisites

Exercises you need to master prior to performing this exercise:

> Core breath (p. 81)
>
> Squat (p. 86)
>
> Standing one-leg transfer (p. 89)
>
> Lunge (p. 90)
>
> Monster walk (p. 184)
>
> Standing biceps curl (p. 128)
>
> Deadlift (p. 174)
>
> Frankenstein walk (p. 177)
>
> Standing upright row with band (p. 151)
>
> Pallof press (p. 100)

Description

- With baby safely in the carrier (see previous exercise), inhale to expand and lower into a squat if your bag is on the floor or any lower surface.
- Exhale to engage your Core 4 as you reach to lift your baby bag and place it on your shoulder.
- Inhale to expand then exhale to engage as you rise out of the squat.
- Adjust the bag onto both shoulders (if you are using a backpack), and center your body so the weight is distributed in a way that you can maintain your alignment.

Safety Considerations

Be sure to follow the directions on your carrier if using one. With a load on your front and on your back, be aware of your posture and alignment. The weights can offset each other, but one may become dominant and force you to lose your neutral spine.

Car Seat Squat

This exercise builds strength and endurance in the legs, trains your glutes and pelvic floor in a very functional way, and prepares you for one of the most common movements of motherhood.

Prerequisites

Exercises you need to master prior to performing this exercise:

> Core breath (p. 81)
>
> Squat (p. 86)
>
> Squat and back row (p. 123)
>
> Standing biceps curl (p.128) or standing hammer curl (p. 131)
>
> Pallof press (p. 100)
>
> Alternating front raise (p. 155)
>
> Upright row (p. 121)
>
> Deadlift (p. 172)
>
> Standing one leg transfer (p. 89)

Equipment

An infant car seat

Description

- Place the car seat on the ground with the carry arm locked upright.
- Stand with feet pelvis-width apart in front of the car seat.
- Inhale to expand as you squat down, using good squat form.
- Grab the carry arm of the car seat with both hands in front of you *(a)*.
- Exhale to engage then press back up to standing while lifting the car seat *(b)*.

Safety Considerations

If you feel any heaviness in your pelvis, start with the car seat on a wide chair so you will not need to go as deep into your squat.

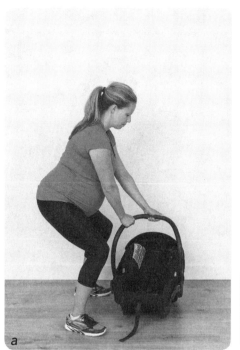 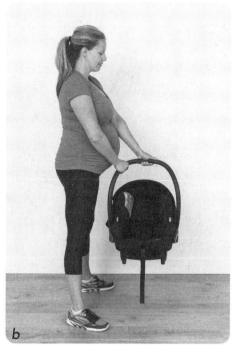

Bucket Car Seat Lift

If you already have your bucket car seat, great! If not, no worries; you can use a duffel bag with some weight in it to start practicing this lift.

Prerequisites

Exercises you need to master prior to performing this exercise:

> Core breath (p. 81)
>
> Squat (p. 86)
>
> Standing one-leg transfer (p. 89)
>
> Pallof press (p. 100)
>
> Seated march on stability ball (p. 88)
>
> Standing hammer curl (p. 131)
>
> Upright row (p. 121)

Description

- Stand with your baby's bucket car seat beside your right leg.
- As you squat down to reach for the bucket, remember to inhale to expand (a).
- Grab the handle, exhale to engage your Core 4, and rise up from your squat while holding the bucket (b) with a slightly bent elbow to engage the biceps (c).
- Repeat as many as you can with great form and then switch sides.

Safety Considerations

Maintain a bent elbow to maximize use of the biceps and minimize the load on the neck muscles, particularly your upper traps. Keep your spine in a neutral position as you squat.

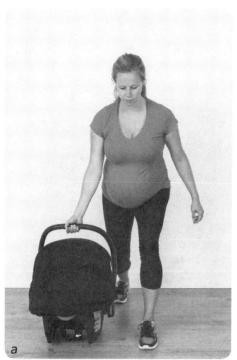

a

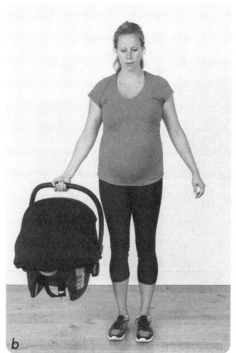

b

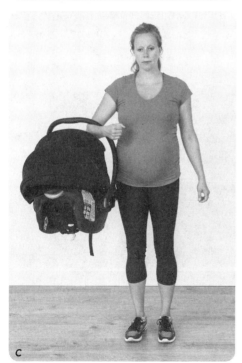

c

Bucket Car Seat Carry

As the Bucket Car Seat Lift exercise becomes easier, you can follow it with this exercise, which adds movement.

Prerequisites

Exercises you need to master prior to performing this exercise:

Core breath (p. 81)

Squat (p. 86)

Standing one-leg transfer (p. 89)

Lunge and one-arm row (p. 125)

Standing biceps curl (p. 128)

Upright row (p. 121)

Description

- Stand with your baby's bucket car seat beside your right leg.
- As you squat down to reach for the bucket, remember to inhale to expand.
- Grab the handle, exhale to engage, and rise up from your squat while holding the bucket with a slightly bent elbow to engage the biceps.
- Once you are standing, practice walking while carrying the bucket. Pay attention to your posture and make sure you are not leaning too far to the side or back.

Safety Considerations

If you are leaning too far to the opposite side or straining to hold the bucket, it is too heavy. Decrease the load until you can maintain proper alignment.

Stroller Fold and Unfold

Every stroller is just a little bit different, but the general movement mechanics that you will engage in are similar.

Prerequisites

Exercises you need to master prior to performing this exercise:

>Core breath (p. 81)
>
>Squat (p. 86)
>
>Lunge (p.90)
>
>Standing hammer curl (p. 128)
>
>Chest press with band (p. 106)
>
>Triceps press with stability ball (p. 142)
>
>Alternating front raise (p. 155)
>
>Upright row (p. 121)
>
>Standing upright row with band (p. 151)

Description

- Stand at the side of the stroller near the release button.
- Hold the handle and press the release.
- Inhale to expand as you lower the handle to fold it.
- Exhale to engage as you return to a standing position, or follow with the Stroller Lift (see next exercise).

Safety Considerations

It will be difficult to maintain a neutral spine here, because you will likely need to squat all the way down. To protect the spine, avoid bending forward from the waist.

Stroller Lift

Now that the stroller is folded, you need to lift it to put it where it needs to go—in the car, in a closet, or up the stairs. Start with just lifting and setting down the stroller. In the next exercise we will show you how to put it into the car.

Prerequisites

Exercises you need to master prior to performing this exercise:

      Core breath (p. 81)

      Squat (p. 86)

      Lunge (p. 90)

      Standing one-leg transfer (p. 89)

      Standing biceps curl (p. 128)

      Chest press with band (p. 106)

      Triceps press with stability ball (p. 142)

      Alternating front raise (p. 155)

      Upright row (p. 121)

      Standing upright row with band (p. 151)

Description

- Start with the Stroller Fold if the stroller is still in the upright position. Or, if the stroller is already folded, then begin with an inhale down into your squat.
- Grab the ends of the stroller, keeping your body parallel to the stroller and maintaining a neutral curve in your lower back (lumbar spine) as much as possible.
- Exhale to engage your Core 4 and rise out of your squat with the stroller in hand.
- Once you are in a standing position, inhale and then exhale to place the stroller on the surface you have chosen, or follow with the Stroller Lift Into Car (see next exercise).

Safety Considerations

Protecting your back during this lift is critical. Many things are working against your lower-back stability—the increase in relaxin, fatigue, poor alignment, increased flexion load while nursing, loss of abdominal control and support. Therefore, lifting a 20-pound (9 kg) stroller is not easy on the spine. It is critical that you keep as close to a neutral arch as possible during the lift.

Stroller Lift Into Car

Now that you are good at maneuvering the stroller, it is time to practice getting it into and out of the trunk of the car. It is very difficult to do this with perfect ergonomics. Hatchbacks will be a little easier to work with than sedans. The trick to putting a stroller into the trunk of the car is using as much of your body mechanics as possible while avoiding twisting.

Prerequisites

Exercises you need to master prior to performing this exercise:

Core breath (p. 81)

Squat (p. 86)

Lunge (p. 90)

Deadlift (p. 172)

Standing one-leg transfer (p. 89)

Standing biceps curl (p. 128)

Chest press with band (p. 106)

Triceps press with stability ball (p. 142)

Upright row (p. 121)

Standing upright row with band (p. 151)

Description

- If you have just completed the Stroller Lift, then take your inhale to reset, exhale to engage the Core 4 again, and step forward into a lunge with your lead leg closer to the trunk.
- As your body weight comes forward onto the lead leg, use the momentum to thrust the stroller into the trunk.
- Feel free to rest the stroller on the edge of the trunk to get yourself positioned correctly.
- You will need to lower into a more asymmetrical squat to gently place the stroller into the trunk.
- For lower cars, use a deadlift by inhaling to expand, exhale to engage, and hinge forward at the hips, keeping the stroller as close to you as possible as you lower it into the trunk.

Safety Considerations

Remember to keep a neutral spine during this exercise to protect your spine.

Stroller Lift Out of Car

Getting the stroller out of the car will also take some practice. To lift a stroller out of the trunk, you will need to reverse the Stroller Lift Into Car to some degree.

Prerequisites

Exercises you need to master prior to performing this exercise:

Core breath (p. 81)

Squat (p. 86)

Lunge (p. 90)

Deadlift (p. 172)

Standing one-leg transfer (p. 89)

Standing biceps curl (p. 128)

Chest press with band (p. 106)

Triceps press with stability ball (p. 142)

Upright row (p. 121)

Standing upright row with band (p. 151)

Description

- Stand facing the trunk in a lunge position with your back foot facing where you are going to put the stroller down.
- Inhale down into the lunge as you reach for the stroller.
- Exhale and engage as you pick up the stroller and move your weight onto your back foot.
- Feel free to rest the stroller on the edge of the trunk.
- Bring your leg closest to the trunk toward the other leg. Inhale down into a squat to place the stroller on the ground.
- If you find the stroller too heavy to use for practice, start with some sandbag weights or a heavy duffle bag.
- For lower cars, you can also use a deadlift to remove the stroller by inhaling and hinging forward at the hips to grasp the stroller. Then, exhale to engage and use your glutes and arm strength to lift the stroller out of the trunk.

Safety Considerations

- Remember to keep a neutral spine during this exercise to protect your spine.
- Exhale on every exertion to engage your Core 4.
- Getting a stroller out of the trunk is a very difficult task. Go easy and build yourself up to being able to handle the awkward size of the stroller by starting with smaller items like golf umbrellas, umbrella strollers, and fold-up shopping carts. Also, be sure the stroller is locked in the folded position when you are lifting it.

Stroller Carry

Stairs are a part of daily life and you may need to navigate stairs with your stroller. Subways and buses in most cities are getting better about strollers, but there will always be a few stairs, perhaps even to get into and out of your own home!

Prerequisites

Exercises you need to master prior to performing this exercise:

Core breath (p. 81)

Standing one-leg transfer (p. 89)

Lunge (p. 90)

Squat and back row (p. 123)

Monster walk (p. 184)

Standing biceps curl (p. 128)

Description

- Inhale to expand and lower into a squat.
- Exhale to engage, grab the ends of the stroller, and lift with your Core 4 engaged.
- Continue to inhale and exhale as you go up the stairs. Your Core 4 will not and should not fully release, but the tension will wax and wane, and should not be held braced.

Safety Considerations

As with the other stroller exercises, be mindful of your spine. Start with something lighter and build up your strength if you are losing form or not feeling particularly strong on a certain day. Strollers are awkward, but you may be carrying one with a sleeping baby in it very soon!

Baby Into Bucket

Getting your baby into and out of the car seat requires a lot of flexibility and balance. Typically, you will set the car seat on the floor before placing your baby in it so it doesn't accidentally fall off a higher surface with your baby inside.

Prerequisites

Exercises you need to master prior to performing this exercise:

> Core breath (p. 81)
>
> Squat (p. 86)
>
> Squat and back row (p. 123)
>
> Standing one-leg transfer (p. 89)
>
> Lunge (p. 90)
>
> One-arm bent-over row (p. 118)
>
> Standing biceps curl (p. 128)
>
> Deadlift (p. 172)
>
> Standing upright row with band (p. 151)

Description

- Stand directly in front of the car seat.
- Inhale down into a deep squat while holding the "practice baby" (you can use a weight or sandbag to practice, starting light with about five pounds (2 kg) and increasing to 10 to 15 pounds (4.5 to 7 kg) as you get stronger and more flexible).
- Exhale to engage your pelvic floor and extend your arms to lower the baby into the bucket.
- Inhale and exhale normally as you attach the safety belts.
- Inhale to expand and exhale to engage your pelvic floor and rise out of the squat.

Safety Considerations

Whenever you go to pick up your baby, even when just practicing, remember to use core breath to engage the Core 4.

Bucket Into Car

The bucket is a tricky little thing. Heavy and awkward by itself, when you add in your most precious cargo it takes on a life of its own! To get the bucket into the car requires a lift and a twist. This is best to practice without any weight at first to get the movement down right.

Prerequisites

Exercises you need to master prior to performing this exercise:

Core breath (p. 81)

Squat (p. 86)

Standing one-leg transfer (p. 89)

Lunge (p. 90)

Monster walk (p. 184)

Standing biceps curl (p. 128)

Deadlift (p. 172)

Standing upright row with band (p. 151)

Pallof press (p. 100)

Description

- If the bucket is on the ground, start with the Bucket Lift.
- Using core breath, inhale to expand and exhale to engage as you move into a semilunge position with your right leg closer to the open door, or even inside the car.
- Take a moment to inhale, then exhale to thrust the bucket into the car and onto the seat.
- Slide and wiggle the bucket until it lands perfectly on the locking mechanism. If it is stiff or difficult to move, pause and inhale again and then use your exhale to give your body the stability it needs to work the bucket into position. This will help prevent excessive loads on your spine.
- Once the bucket is locked in, inhale again, then exhale to engage your core to get out of the car.

Safety Considerations

This exercise can become more and more difficult as your belly grows. Be mindful of not creating too much intra-abdominal pressure as you struggle to get the bucket into the car and attached to the locking mechanism. Take your time to master the movements and feel free to rest the bucket on the seat as you reset yourself to exhale and engage.

Bucket Out of Car

If there is one thing you will do a lot, you will put your baby into and take your baby out of the car. Sometimes, you will take your baby out and then take the car seat out later. Other times, your baby will be sleeping, and you will not want to disturb your baby, so you will need to put the bucket seat with your baby in it into the car and take it out of the car. This exercise is meant to train you in the awkward movement and positions ahead of time.

Prerequisites

Exercises you need to master prior to performing this exercise:

> Core breath (p. 81)
>
> Squat (p. 86)
>
> Standing one-leg transfer (p. 89)
>
> Lunge (p. 90)
>
> Lunge with one-arm row (p. 125)
>
> Standing biceps curl (p. 128)
>
> One-leg deadlift (p. 182)
>
> Standing upright row with band (p. 151)
>
> Pallof press (p. 100)

Description

- Stand next to the open car door.
- Inhale to expand and exhale to engage and lunge your right foot into the right passenger side, or you can use the bottom of the door opening to give you leverage.
- Reach and unlock the bucket.
- Inhale to expand and exhale to engage as you lift the bucket off the mechanism and lunge back into the starting standing position.

Safety Considerations

This exercise, like the previous one, can become more and more difficult as your belly grows. Be mindful of not creating too much intra-abdominal pressure as you struggle to get the bucket unlocked and lifted. Take your time to master the movements and feel free to rest the bucket on the seat as you reset yourself to exhale and engage.

Bucket Swing

Sometimes you will put your baby in the bucket car seat but not be quite ready to put her or him in the car (remember, never leave your baby alone in the car, even secured in the bucket). While baby waits, he or she may fuss a bit and can be soothed with some swinging of the bucket car seat.

Prerequisites

Exercises you need to master prior to performing this exercise:

> Core breath (p. 81)
>
> Squat (p. 86)
>
> Deadlift (p. 172)
>
> Standing one-leg transfer (p. 89)
>
> Monster walk (p. 184)
>
> Frankenstein walk (p. 176)
>
> Standing biceps curl (p. 128)
>
> Upright row (p. 121)

Description

- Follow the instruction for the Bucket Car Seat Lift exercise earlier in the chapter.

- Hook one arm under the handle and have the bucket close in to your body or hold the handle with both hands and arms straight (this can be more challenging to your lower back so be careful). Pay attention to your posture and try not to lean back.

- You can plant your feet and swing your arms or step side to side or front to back while hanging on to the bucket.

Safety Considerations

Always be mindful of things around you so you don't knock baby into a wall, piece of furniture, or another child. Maintain good posture with this one, because the bucket plus your baby is quite a load. And watch that you don't hold your breath, which increases your intra-abdominal pressure.

Baby Wearing

Wearing a baby involves a lot of endurance and postural control. If you do not already have a baby carrier, then wearing a backpack on your front can help prepare you. With the added weight forward, you will have a tendency in the earlier part of your pregnancy to lean back and tuck your bum, which is not optimal (see photo *b*). This exercise is designed to help you avoid that posture, become aware of your body position, and strengthen your core so you can stand well aligned while carrying your baby (see photo *a*). Start with about five pounds (2 kg) and work your way up to 10 to 15 pounds (4.5 to 7 kg). You can use a sandbag, weights, or a small bag of dog food to be your "baby."

Prerequisites

Exercises you need to master prior to performing this exercise:

> Core breath (p. 81)
>
> Standing one-leg transfer (p. 89)
>
> Squat (p. 86)
>
> Monster walk (p. 184)
>
> Bird dog (p. 96)
>
> Side knee plank (p. 94)
>
> Lunge with biceps curl (p. 136)

Description

- Put on your baby carrier or sling or wear a backpack on your front.
- Now practice standing in place, stepping side to side, or walking with the baby in your front carrier.
- Now, try squatting. If you are not already holding your "practice baby," remember to line yourself up square to the baby before squatting to lift it.
- Inhale to expand as you lower down into a squat.
- Exhale to engage as you pick up the baby and rise to standing.
- Start with wearing baby for just a few minutes or until you lose form. Build your tolerance up to 15 to 20 minutes. You can even take the baby for a walk around the neighborhood!

Safety Considerations

Be mindful of your posture and do *not* tuck your bum once you are standing. Tucking your bum under will minimize your use of your glutes and pelvic floor muscles and force the obliques and hip flexors to overcompensate.

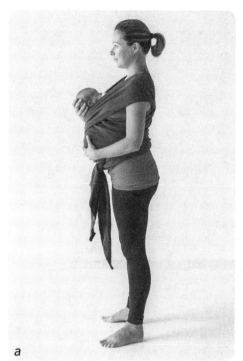

a

Courtesy of Jenn Di Spirito.

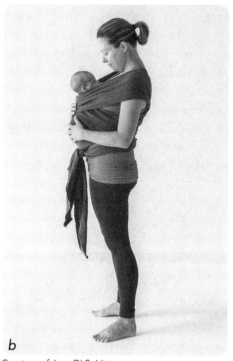

b

Courtesy of Jenn Di Spirito.

This is one of the most difficult movements to do with good form, especially when you have a real baby who is sleeping whom you don't want to wake! But here is how you can best prepare your body for the load.

Prerequisites

Exercises you need to master prior to performing this exercise:

Core breath (p. 81)

Squat (p. 86)

Lunge (p. 90)

Deadlift (p. 172)

Standing one-leg transfer (p. 89)

Standing biceps curl (p. 128)

Chest press with band (p. 106)

Triceps press with stability ball (p. 142)

Upright row (p. 121)

Standing upright row with band (p. 151)

Pallof press (p. 100)

Description

- First, practice without holding any weight, then use something very light, gradually adding more weight as you get comfortable with the movement.
- If the side rails of the crib go down, then place them in the lowest position.
- You can start to practice with the mattress at the highest position, then gradually lower its position as you master this movement.
- For ease of demonstrating the movement, we chose a chair to act as the crib. If you already have a crib, then it is best to practice with the real thing. If you have yet to purchase a crib, then using a chair as shown is a great way to mimic the movement (a and b).
- Stand facing the side of the crib and holding the "practice baby" close to your body in front of you (a).
- Inhale to expand and prepare.
- Exhale to engage and hinge forward at the hip, keeping the baby close in to you.
- When the side rail limits your descent, lower your arms toward the mattress as much as possible (b).
- Set the baby on the mattress as gently as possible.
- Keep the core engaged, take a small breath in, then exhale as you straighten back up.

Safety Considerations

Ergonomics are tough to maintain here, but do your best. Be mindful not to hold your breath, because this will increase your intra-abdominal pressure. Try to keep a neutral spine as long as you can.

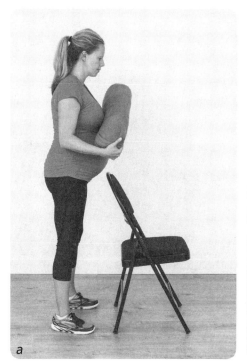
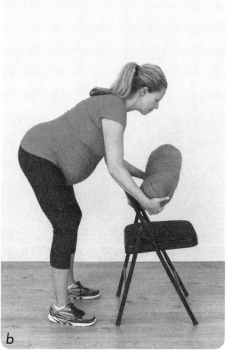

Lift Baby Out of Crib

This is one of the most difficult movements to do. It is nearly impossible for the average mom to lift a baby out of the crib with perfect ergonomics due to the safety design of the crib. Maintaining a neutral spine is difficult due to the height of the railings and mattress in relation to your height. But here is how you can best prepare your body for the load.

Prerequisites

Exercises you need to master prior to performing this exercise:

Core breath (p. 81)

Squat (p. 86)

Lunge (p. 90)

Deadlift and back row (p. 174)

One-leg deadlift (p. 182)

Standing one-leg transfer (p. 89)

Standing biceps curl (p. 128)

Chest press with band (p. 106)

Triceps press with stability ball (p. 142)

Upright row (p. 121)

Standing upright row with band (p. 151)

Description

- First practice without lifting any weight. Then, use something very light, gradually adding more weight as you get comfortable with the movement.
- Stand facing the baby in the crib. Inhale to expand as you hinge at the hips and extend your arms over the side of the crib to the baby.
- Exhale to engage as you scoop the baby up.
- Bring the baby close to your chest as you try to maintain a neutral spine, squeeze your glutes, and return to a standing position.

Safety Considerations

Ergonomics are tough to maintain here, but do your best. Again, be mindful not to hold your breath as this will increase your intra-abdominal pressure. Resume proper alignment as soon as you have completely straightened up to help minimize the load on the spine.

Standing Baby Rocks

Babies like to be soothed by being held and rocked. You can do this seated (see the next exercise, Seated Baby Rocks) or you can do it standing. Add a little music and you can even turn it into a slow dance, which will often be the case when you are out running errands with your baby. Remember, never, ever leave your baby alone in the car, even for a few minutes!

Prerequisites

Exercises you need to master prior to performing this exercise:

Squat (p. 86)

Lunge (p. 90)

Monster walk (p. 184)

Standing one-leg transfer (p. 89)

Standing biceps curl (p. 128)

Frankenstein walk (p. 176)

Alternating front raise (p. 155)

Description

- Stand with your feet pelvis-width apart. Whether your baby is in your arms or a carrier, keep your ribs over your pelvis and your pelvis in a neutral position.
- Transfer your weight from side to side as you rock or put one foot forward and transfer your weight from front to back.
- Try making figure eights with your pelvis, allowing your pelvis to move in and out of neutral. Be sure to come back to neutral position at the end of this movement.

Safety Considerations

When you are standing, especially when carrying a load, it is important to pay attention to your posture. The weight of your baby will draw you forward and cause you to tuck your bum under and thrust your ribs up, effectively taking the pelvic floor and glutes out of this exercise.

Babies like to be soothed by being held and rocked. As we learned in the previous exercise, this can be done from a standing position. It can also be done from a seated position on a stability ball, which is a nice movement for you and provides gentle bouncing for your baby.

Prerequisites

Exercises you need to master prior to performing this exercise:

Squat (p. 86)

Lunge (p. 90)

Monster walk (p. 184)

Standing one-leg transfer (p. 89)

Standing biceps curl (p. 106)

Description

- With your baby in a carrier or held securely with one arm, use your free hand to stabilize the stability ball.
- Inhale to expand and lower yourself into a squat to sit on your ball.
- Be sure to adjust your posture so your ribs are over your pelvis and you are sitting on your sitz bones.
- Gently and carefully, especially if you and your baby are new to this, move around on the ball: bounce up and down, rock side to side, rock forward and back.
- You can do figure-8s once you have mastered the rocking.
- You can add the core breath by slowing down the movement and inhaling to expand, then exhaling to engage the Core 4 as you move away from the center of balance.
- Once your baby is soothed and it is time to get up, inhale to expand then exhale to engage your Core 4 as you rise up off the ball. You may need one hand on the ball to stabilize it as you rise.

Safety Considerations

If you are not used to using the stability ball or don't feel securely balanced on it yet, start with the ball in the corner of the room, propped up against the two walls. A wider foot stance will also increase the stability while working on the ball.

Laundry Squat

You will not believe how much laundry one little person can generate in a 24-hour period. You will be doing *a lot* of laundry! And with lots of laundry comes lots of lifting and carrying of awkward laundry baskets up and down stairs. With the higher levels of the hormone relaxin in your body for many more months, it's important to move properly while lifting and carrying to prevent unwanted injury.

Prerequisites

Exercises you need to master prior to performing this exercise:

> Core breath (p. 81)
>
> Squat (p. 86)
>
> Deadlift (p. 172)
>
> Standing one-leg transfer (p. 89)
>
> Standing biceps curl (p. 128)
>
> Alternating front raise (p. 155)
>
> Upright row (p. 121)
>
> Standing upright row with band (p. 151)

Description

Every time you pick up a laundry basket you can use a deadlift or a squat. Squatting is the first choice and can also be used when folding laundry, especially if you have a front-load dryer.

Squat to Pick Up Basket

- Stand with your feet hip-width or a little wider apart in front of your laundry basket.
- Inhale to expand as you squat to lower down, then exhale to engage the Core 4 and lift your basket.
- You can carry the basket in front of you, tight to your body with both hands, or you may rest it on a hip while you walk.
- If you carry the basket on one hip, switch sides each time you do your laundry.

Deadlift to Pick Up Basket

Use the same steps as for the Squat to Pick Up Basket, but instead of lowering into a squat, hinge the hips and bend forward to pick up the basket. This movement will place more strain on your lower back than squatting will, so use it only for lighter loads.

- Stand with your feet hip-width or a little wider apart, in front of your laundry basket.
- Inhale to expand as you slide your hand down the front of your legs and reach for the basket, keeping your spine neutral.

(continued)

- Exhale to engage the Core 4 and lift your basket. Use your glutes to pull you back up to standing.
- You can carry the basket in front of you, tight to your body with both hands, or you may rest it on a hip while you walk. If you carry the basket on one hip, switch sides each time you do your laundry.

Squat to Fold Laundry

- Inhale as you squat to lower down and grab your piece of laundry.
- Exhale to engage the Core 4 and press back up.

Safety Considerations

Be mindful of how much weight you are lifting in the baskets. It is better to do multiple trips as you build your strength. You can even start with an empty basket to master the movement incorporating the core breath.

You can see how many of these movements for motherhood require the same sort of strengthening exercises, and the one thing they all have in common is using the core breath to engage the pelvic floor and Core 4. The core breath sets up a stable base, which provides leverage during the hard (heavy or awkward) part of the movement. Just like in regular fitness training, you exhale on the hard part. It is the same with movements in motherhood, but now you are more aware of why you exhale—to get the Core 4 working for you!

Sample Programs for Each Phase of Pregnancy

10

Choosing Your Program and Level of Fitness

There is no question that exercise is a fundamental part of a healthy lifestyle. The benefits far outweigh the risks, and this does not change once you become pregnant. However, you do have to be smart and listen to your body (just like you would before pregnancy), because the many physical and physiological changes that occur from the moment you conceive until the birth of your baby can certainly change your focus and how you work out.

If you are having a safe, uncomplicated pregnancy, you are encouraged to exercise to ensure your body maintains optimal fitness and health and is ready to manage the demands of labor, birth, and motherhood (Davies et al. 2003). One thing we have always said and truly live by is, if there is ever a time in your life to exercise, it is during pregnancy! You are creating a life and that life is completely dependent on you. You are also facing one of the most physically and mentally demanding events you will ever endure, so you need to train to make sure you are fit for birth. In fact, it is considered a risk factor to *not* exercise during pregnancy (Wolfe and Mottola 2000).

Pregnancy can present a few challenges for some and many challenges for others, but many of these challenges can be minimized or avoided by having a strong and healthy body. The American Congress of Gynecologists and Obstetricians (ACOG) and the Society of Obstetricians and Gynecologists of Canada (SOGC) recommend strength training, partnered with flexibility and cardiovascular exercise most days of the week (American Congress of Gynecologists and Obstetricians 2015; Society of Obstetricians and Gynecologists of Canada 2003). This book follows those guidelines and gives you the specific exercises that will prepare your body for labor and birth as well as motherhood.

RISKS AND CONTRAINDICATIONS TO EXERCISE IN PREGNANCY

In this section we will outline the risks and warning signs to watch out for when it comes to exercise during pregnancy. It is important to listen to your body and pay attention to your response during exercise to tell whether you should modify your activity or stop it altogether to avoid injury.

As your belly grows, it is recommended that at 16 weeks gestation all back-lying exercises be modified to an incline position (think heart above baby) so as not to put additional pressure on the inferior vena cava, a large vein that returns blood flow back to the heart from the lower half of the body. However, some women have no problem lying on their back, so listen to *your* body and respond to what it is telling you.

Maternal heart rate increases approximately 10 to 15 beats per minute (Brown 2016), but keep in mind that each individual adapts to exercise differently. An Olympic athlete, a fitness enthusiast, and a sedentary person all have different resting heart rates and levels of intensity that can be maintained within healthy limits (we will cover this in more detail later in this chapter). This is why it is important to always listen to your body, speak with your healthcare provider, and ensure that exercise during pregnancy is specific to the event you are training for—labor and birth. Although you want to be aware of the published guidelines, note that SOGC has updated the heart rate guidelines and, as of December 2015, ACOG no longer uses heart rate as a measurement of exertion (American Congress of Obstetricians and Gynecologists 2017).

As mentioned previously, exercising during pregnancy is an excellent practice for most women. However, there are conditions that you may suffer from before becoming pregnant or may develop during your pregnancy that can affect whether or not you should exercise. Table 10.1 provides contraindications for exercise in pregnancy and tables 10.2 and 10.3 provide contraindications for aerobic exercise in pregnancy.

Table 10.1 Contraindications to Exercise During Pregnancy: Questions to Discuss with Your Physician When Considering an Exercise Program During Pregnancy

Have you developed any of the following pregnancy-related conditions?

- Premature labor
- Ruptured membranes (rupture of the amniotic sac (bag) that surrounds the fetus)
- Persistent bleeding during the second or third trimester, or placenta previa (where the placenta grows in the uterus covering all or part of the opening to the cervix)
- Pregnancy-induced high blood pressure (or preeclampsia)
- Incompetent cervix (a condition where the cervix widens and thins before the end of the pregnancy)
- Evidence of poor growth of the fetus while in the womb (referred to as intrauterine growth restriction), or you are carrying more than one fetus

Have you experienced any of the following conditions?

- A history of miscarriage or premature labor in previous pregnancies
- Anemia or low iron (iron deficiency): your physician will often describe anemia as a decrease in the number of red blood cells or a less than normal quantity of hemoglobin (that is, a concentration of less than 100 g/L) in your blood
- Malnutrition (an unbalanced diet where certain nutrients are missing) or an eating disorder (such as anorexia, bulimia)
- Any other significant medical condition

Source: Electronic Physical Activity Readiness Medial Examination (ePARmedX-+). Available: http://eparamedx.com, Reprinted with permission of the PAR-Q+ Collaboration.

Table 10.2 Absolute Contraindications to Aerobic Exercise During Pregnancy.

Absolute contraindications

- Hemodynamically significant heart disease
- Restrictive lung disease
- Incompetent cervix or cerclage
- Multiple gestation at risk for premature labor
- Persistent bleeding in second or third trimester
- Placenta previa after 26 weeks gestation
- Premature labor in current pregnancy
- Ruptured membranes
- Preeclampsia or pregnancy-induced hypertension
- Severe anemia

Reprinted with permission from Physical activity and exercise during pregnancy and the postpartum period. Committee Opinion No. 650. American College of Obstetricians and Gynecologists. *Obstet Gynecol* 2015: 126: e135-42.

Table 10.3 Relative Contraindications to Aerobic Exercise During Pregnancy

Relative contraindications	
• Anemia • Unelevated maternal cardiac arrhythmia • Chronic bronchitis • Poorly controlled type I diabetes • Extreme morbid obesity • History of extremely sedentary lifestyle	• Intrauterine growth restriction in current pregnancy • Poorly controlled hypertension • Orthopedic limitations • Poorly controlled seizure disorder • Poorly controlled hyperthyroidism • Heavy smoker

Reprinted with permission from Physical activity and exercise during pregnancy and the postpartum period. Committee Opinion No. 650. American College of Obstetricians and Gynecologists. *Obstet Gynecol* 2015: 126: e135-42.

Along with those from tables 10.1, 10.2, and 10.3, other risk factors include the following:

- Gestational diabetes
- High blood pressure
- Toxemia
- Varicose veins
- Excessive weight gain
- Back pain
- Edema

EXERCISE GOALS DURING PREGNANCY

Exercising during pregnancy should be adapted as necessary to ensure you and your baby's health and safety, and that you feel good while exercising throughout all trimesters. Just like you would when you are not pregnant, follow the necessary precautions, start at your current fitness level or even go a little easier, and listen to your body.

The exercise workouts are designed for three different levels of exerciser. Here is a quick description of beginner to advanced exercisers:

- *Beginner:* A beginner exerciser is someone who has not been exercising or who exercises sporadically with little knowledge or expertise regarding fitness and exercise programming. She is uncertain about what exercises she can or cannot do and often feels intimidated about going to the gym. She struggles with maintaining a regular exercise routine and needs constant support and guidance.

- *Intermediate:* An intermediate exerciser is someone who regularly exercises two to three times per week with a good understanding of fitness for health and body composition. She feels confident in the gym and tries a variety of different exercise routines and techniques. She enjoys fitness and understands it's a part of her healthy lifestyle.

- *Advanced:* An advanced exerciser is someone who has extensive knowledge of fitness and exercise programming and who exercises four to five times per week at higher intensities. She is open to new challenges and likes to push herself to new heights. Barring complications, she will eagerly continue to exercise right through her pregnancy and will already have a plan in place for getting back into the gym after birth.

Exercising during pregnancy should have four main goals:

1. Maintain (or if you are previously sedentary, gain) strength, mobility, and cardiovascular health.
2. Connect and train the inner core system.
3. Move in ways that optimize posture and alignment.
4. Train the body for labor, birth and recovery.

When you follow an exercise program it is important to make sure that the above goals are covered throughout all three trimesters as well as during your recovery. This is *not* the time to train for a triathlon or improve your one rep max. Instead, you want to train for your birth marathon and ensure you are giving yourself all the benefits of a strong and healthy body and, in turn, a head start for your recovery. Research has proven that muscle does have memory and the stronger and healthier you are during your pregnancy, the better your recovery experience will be (Bruusgaard, Johansen, Engner, Rana, and Gundersen 2010). Remember this protocol for your pregnancy, birth, and recovery:

- *Train* during your pregnancy.
- *Recover and retrain* after birth.
- *Restore* beyond the first eight weeks postpartum.

Train

During each trimester, the focus always stays the same in that you want to optimize and support the physical and physiological changes that are occurring as each month passes. You also want to pay attention to the signs and symptoms that may be telling you to either amp it up a little bit or scale back.

Exercise during pregnancy should still follow the same protocols as if you weren't pregnant. The "FITT" formula is a great way to outline your exercise regimen. FITT stands for Frequency, Intensity, Time, and Type: let's take a look at each component.

Frequency

Work out three to five times per week depending on your fitness level. Beginners will start with two to three times per week and increase frequency as they gain strength and endurance. Your goal is to exercise regularly most days of the week.

Intensity

Work at an intensity measured on a RPE scale from 1 to 10 (see table 1.1 in chapter 1). It is not based on heart rate, but rather on your own rate of perceived exertion. The goal for all pregnant women is to work at a level of 4 (somewhat hard) throughout their routine. You want to finish feeling like you had a good workout but are not exhausted (Austin and Seebohar 2011).

To gauge this, remember to not run out of breath. It is important to be able to carry on a short conversation without gasping for air or sweating profusely. Also remember that your heart rate increases approximately 10 beats per minute as a result of pregnancy, so it may take a little time for you to adapt to these changes when you begin to exercise. Take it slow and progress at your own comfort level to ensure that the above guidelines are met. Figure 10.1 shows heart rate guidelines for exercise during pregnancy.

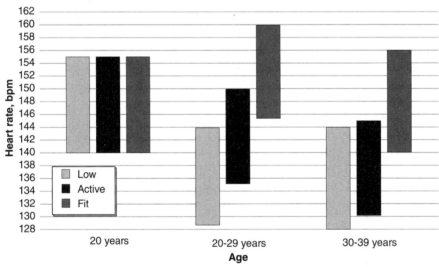

Data from Mottola et al. 2006, Davenport et al. 2008.

Figure 10.1   Suggested Heart Rate Guidelines for Exercise During Pregnancy

Note: The above guidelines are from the SOGC and the Canadian Society for Exercise Physiology and are quite conservative. You will also notice that there is no heart rate guideline for women in their 40s. More and more women are getting pregnant later in life and exercise should still be supported, so we encourage you to get clearance from your doctor.

Time

Beginners should start with 15 minutes of continuous cardiovascular activity two to three times a week, adding two to three minutes per week to a maximum of 30 to 40 minutes, three to five times per week. Strength training would fall within the same guidelines of time. Remember, though, there are exceptions to every rule. Listen to your body! If it doesn't feel right, don't do it. During pregnancy, each day can feel different from the next. What you may not be able to do today may be much easier tomorrow, and what you are able to do today you may not be able to do tomorrow. So always listen to your body.

Type

When strength training, perform exercises that use the largest muscles first. This helps you maintain stamina throughout the workout. If you strength-train three days per week, a full-body routine is recommended for each session with at least one day in between for rest. If you strength train four or more days per week, you can do a split routine on alternate days; that is, do your upper-body routine one day and your lower-body routine the next. This way you follow the rule of resting between muscle groups. Always ensure to include some cardiovascular training most days of the week. Remember, the Core 4 are always working even while strength training. Pay special attention to core stability, posture, and supporting structures (abdominals, upper and lower back, triceps, and glutes) while strength training.

Beginners should perform one to two sets of 8 to 12 repetitions with one- to two-minute rest periods between sets. Intermediate and advanced exercisers should perform two to three sets of 12 or more repetitions with 1 minute of rest between sets. In addition, the general rest/recovery rule for pregnancy is that you rest for one hour per every hour of activity.

Light-weight-bearing, non-weight-bearing, and low-impact cardiovascular exercises (swimming, stationary cycling, aquatics, walking, using an elliptical machine) are recommended for beginners. Intermediate and advanced exercisers can continue with their regular cardiovascular exercise routine as long as they have received clearance from their doctor or midwife. Note that it is recommended to avoid any sports or activities that could possibly cause abdominal trauma or harm the fetus, such as contact sports, high-altitude training, hot yoga, or hot Pilates. We also recommend that high-impact activities like running and jumping be scaled back or ideally avoided after the first trimester to protect the pelvic floor from additional strain.

Exercise Guidelines by Trimester

These basic training guidelines are good to follow during each trimester:

First Trimester

The first trimester is very taxing on your body. Critical development is taking place, so it is important to not overexert yourself or get overheated. You may experience a high degree of fatigue and nausea, which will limit your activity and determine how far you should go. For beginners, start slow with regular walking and build intensity as your comfort level allows.

Second Trimester

The second trimester is when most pregnant women feel "normal." Blood volume catches up to the vasodilation of the blood vessels, so you won't feel as lightheaded and sluggish (Soma-Pillay, Catherine, Tolppanen, Mebazaa, Tolppanen, and Mebazaa 2016).

  Your body has had time to adapt to all the physiological changes that have taken place and you can breathe with ease. However, at around weeks 16 to 20, due to the weight of the uterus on the inferior vena cava, it is recommended to stop exercising while lying on your back. Modify these exercises so you are in an incline position, seated, or standing. Due to the extra weight on the pelvic floor, runners should now change to walking on an incline, using an elliptical machine, or using a stair climber.

Third Trimester

Intensity and duration should not be increased in the third trimester. This is when you find you will naturally slow down. Listen to your body and adjust weights and aerobic activity accordingly. Changing to non-weight-bearing activity (swimming, stationary cycling) is also recommended if you cannot maintain your previous routine comfortably. Now is the time to place extra focus on posture, flexibility, relaxation, and mentally preparing for labor and birth. It is like tapering before race day.

Recover and Retrain

After pregnancy and birth, the abdominal wall has been stretched well beyond the optimal length and, in the case of a cesarean birth, many tissues have been cut as well. Research supports wearing an abdominal wrap (discussed in chapter 4) to help support your pelvis and abdominal wall after a cesarean birth, which is considered major abdominal surgery (Cheifetz, Lucy, Overend, and Crowe 2010). Wearing an abdominal wrap is also a recommended practice if you have a vaginal birth (Litos 2014). In both situations the goal is the same—to provide external support to the tissues that have been stretched, compressed, and maybe even cut, while internal support is retrained with restorative exercise.

The first eight weeks postpartum have been shown to be the time when the most spontaneous healing of the abdominal wall is taking place (Coldron, Stokes, Newham, and Cook 2008). During these first eight weeks, the focus is on reconnecting with the Core 4 and retraining the system to work synergistically. The restorative exercises outlined in chapter 6 are the main focus. Strength training should be avoided until your core function has been restored and a pelvic floor physiotherapist has cleared you to resume exercising (this will be well beyond six weeks postpartum). It is best to begin with cardiovascular training such as short walks around two weeks postpartum and slowly increase your endurance. Listen to your body and make sure there is no pain or pressure on your pelvic floor.

Pregnancy and birth are probably the most physically and physiologically taxing events you will ever experience. During the postpartum period, it is very important to respect your body and honor its accomplishments. Asking for and accepting help so you can focus on healing and rest will assist in your recovery. It is not a sign of weakness. Disregard the "supermom" mentality that is portrayed in the media and instead trust the healing practices of other cultures that emphasize rest, recovery, and being supported, nurtured, and nourished. Having and using support will allow you to focus on resting, recovering, and bonding with your new baby.

After a few weeks, getting outside for short 5-10 minute walks is encouraged as long as you are not experiencing pain, abnormal bleeding, or excessive fatigue. However, use caution because hormones are still elevated and adrenaline can give you a false sense of energy and strength (almost euphoric). Use this time to get outside, enjoy the fresh air and do something for yourself.

The first eight weeks postpartum are truly a time to rest, recover, and retrain. Core breathing, gentle restorative exercises, and reconnecting with your pelvic floor should be among your main priorities.

Pelvic floor physiotherapy is a key part of your recovery. See a physiotherapist between six and eight weeks postpartum (we recommend prebooking this appointment while you are still pregnant) and begin the process of restoring your core. The physiotherapist will monitor your progress (and chances are will commend you for having trained for birth and done your retraining exercises) and will let you know when you have recovered enough to begin restoring your pre-pregnancy fitness level.

Restore

When considering going back to your exercise program, take a breath and think it through. Remember what you just did. You gained 25 to 40 or more pounds (11 to 18 kg), your core muscles were stretched beyond their optimal length, your joints were stressed, your organs may have shifted, *and* you either pushed that baby out or you had major abdominal surgery.

It is monumental! Take time to recover. We cannot stress that enough. In our fast-paced society, we celebrate women who get back in the gym at two weeks postpartum. We invite you to take a different approach. Take time to rest, heal, and retrain your core, and then go back to the gym to work on core restoration and eventually get back to your regular training. The 6- week green light is, in our opinion, irresponsible. Returning to 'normal' activities may take 4, 6, or even 12 months. Everyone is different. It's not a race, and recovery is essential.

Beyond eight weeks postpartum is the time to turn your focus to restoring your core. You have taken time to recover, rest, and retrain. Now it is time to progress the retraining exercises and start to reincorporate strength training and cardio beyond short walks. We recommend you keep the principle of specificity in mind here. Train your body for motherhood. Life as a mom is busy and demanding and you will be moving a lot! Make sure your workouts prepare you for the demands of motherhood.

All in all, exercising during pregnancy and the early stages of the postpartum period should feel good and help you maintain a healthy weight gain and strong muscles to support your changing body. Exercise also may alleviate many of the common aches and pains that pregnant women suffer from. Remember that the best time to prepare for your recovery is while you are still pregnant, so be smart, be safe, and listen to your body. At the end of the day, trust your gut—you are your own best guide during this time.

First Trimester Workouts

11

The pregnant body undergoes some pretty significant changes in the first trimester, such as an increase in blood volume and the production of the hormone relaxin. Add fluctuating emotions, fatigue, and nausea, and you have what is often a very challenging time for some. Movement and exercise can help lessen the discomfort of some of the early changes, but it is important to pay close attention to how you feel. Respect the changes and the effect they will have on your ability to exercise.

Exercising in the first trimester, especially if you are a regular gym goer or class participant, can be really tough with the nausea and low energy levels. Keep in mind that some exercise is *always* better than none and try not to become discouraged if you can't perform at levels you could prior to conceiving. This is temporary and energy levels usually return in the second trimester. Sometimes a simple walk, while it may not feel as strenuous as the exercise you're used to, can be all you need to increase your energy and lift your spirits. Prenatal yoga classes are also great for freeing the mind, body, and spirit during this often challenging time.

It is important to choose your exercise level based on the number of pregnancies you have had and if you were able to retrain and restore your core in between pregnancies. If you are entering this pregnancy with a core that is already facing some challenges such as back pain, hip pain, or pelvic pain or instability, you will need to pay even closer attention to your movement. Dynamic exercise and high-impact activities such as running may be something you want to avoid right from the start. The effect of relaxin on your muscles, joints, and connective tissue makes your entire body (but mainly your pelvis), a bit more lax and unstable, so it is a good idea to avoid any jarring movements and activities such as heavy weightlifting and running.

The following programs for beginner, intermediate, and advanced exercisers were created to help keep you moving most days of the week with the goal of maintaining your current fitness level as you manage nausea and fatigue.

BEGINNER

A beginner exerciser is someone who has not been exercising or who exercises sporadically with little knowledge or expertise regarding fitness and exercise programming. She is uncertain about what exercises she can or cannot do and often feels intimidated about going to the gym. She struggles with maintaining a regular exercise routine and needs constant support and guidance. See table 11.1 for a sample beginner first trimester workout.

Table 11.1 Beginner First Trimester Workout

Activity	Program design		
Cardio	If walking is your only cardio, then do it three to four days per week for 20 minutes per day, or two to three days per week if you also want to include swimming or Aquafit classes. The first trimester is the time that you are creating a habit for the duration of your pregnancy, and walking is one of the best exercises out there. We even recommend walking while you are in labor, so doing it now will literally train you for the big day. Just be careful not to get overheated.		
Full-body strength training	Do your strength training one to two days per week, performing one to two sets with 8 to 12 reps per set. Choose one of the three workouts provided (A, B, or C) or, for a more individualized approach, choose exercises from each one and create your own workout (just make sure to hit all the major muscle groups—legs, chest, back, arms, core).		
	A	Stability ball squat	p. 162
		Deadlift	p. 172
		Clam shell	p. 84
		Ball squeeze rotation	p. 95
		Seated back row	p. 115
		Barbell biceps curl	p. 132
		Skull crusher	p. 140
		Seated shoulder press	p. 154
		Core breath	p. 81
		Bridge	p. 83
		Cat and cow	p. 93
	B	Stability ball lunge	p. 164
		Standing hamstring curl with stability ball	p. 166
		Wall push-up	p. 104

Activity	Program design		
Full-body strength training	**B**	One-arm bent-over row	p. 118
		Concentration curl	p. 138
		Triceps kickback	p. 141
		Lateral raise	p. 152
		Core breath	p. 81
		Clam shell	p. 84
		Bridge	p. 83
		Cat and cow	p. 93
		Chest press with band	p. 106
		Seated lat pulldown	p. 117
		Standing hammer curl	p. 131
		Triceps kickback	p. 141
		Standing upright row with band	p. 151
		Core breath	p. 81
		Clam shell	p. 84
		Bridge	p. 83
		Cat and cow	p. 93
Functional movement	Functional movements are activities and movements that maintain or improve a person's ability to perform activities of daily living. Trying to incorporate these movements on a daily basis, or at least on most days, will help maintain the strength and endurance needed for labor, birth, and motherhood.		
	Walking: Walk as much as you can, because it helps prepare you for labor and the many walks with the stroller, groceries, laundry, etc.		
	Climbing stairs: If you live in a house or apartment with stairs, climbing stairs will help you better prepare for many trips up and down with baby, laundry, etc.		
	Squatting: Find every opportunity to squat as you go about your day, such as when you lift and lower your laundry basket, when you pick an item off the floor, or when you get an item out of a lower cupboard in the kitchen.		
	Lifting: Performing deadlifts as part of your exercise program strengthens the posterior chain and helps prepare you for picking up the car seat and getting the baby in and out of the crib. Practice placing a yoga bolster into the crib and then picking it back up again. Use your deadlift form to perform the movement.		
	Lunges: These help strengthen your legs for both walking and stairs. Do these two to three days per week, performing one to three sets with 8 to 12 reps per set.		

(continued)

Table 11.1   Beginner First Trimester workout *(continued)*

Activity	Program design	
Release work	Perform release exercises daily, holding for 30 to 60 seconds each. Be cautious about overstretching, because the hormone relaxin can give you a false sense of flexibility.	
	Calf stretch	p. 67
	Hamstring stretch with strap	p. 71
	Seated chest stretch over stability ball	p. 63
	4 Stretch	p. 70

INTERMEDIATE

An intermediate exerciser is someone who regularly exercises two to three times per week with a good understanding of fitness for health and weight management. She feels confident in the gym and tries a variety of different exercise routines and techniques. She enjoys fitness and understands it's a part of her lifestyle. See table 11.2 for a sample intermediate first trimester workout.

Table 11.2 Intermediate First Trimester Workout

Activity	Program design		
Cardio	Ideally, you will walk every day even if you do another form of cardio, but if you can only fit one cardio element in that is fine too. Aim for some form of cardio (hiking, swimming, Aquafit classes, gym activities) and a walk four to five days per week. If walking is your only cardio, then do it four to five days per week for at least 30 minutes per day.		
Full-body strength training	Do your strength training two to three days per week, using free weights and body weight, performing two to three sets with 10 to 12 reps per set. Choose one of the three workouts provided (A, B, or C) or, for a more individualized approach, choose exercises from each one and create your own workout (just make sure to hit all the major muscle groups—legs, chest, back, arms, core).		
	A	Deadlift and back row	p. 174
		Calf raise with stability ball	p. 161
		Push-up	p. 112
		Barbell biceps curl	p. 132
		Side-lying triceps press-up	p. 145
		Seated shoulder press	p. 154
		Seated march on stability ball	p. 88
		Crouching tiger	p. 98
		Side knee plank	p. 94
	B	One-arm bent-over row	p. 118
		Calf raise with stability ball	p. 161
		Kneeling ball squeeze	p. 109
		Standing biceps curl on BOSU	p. 137
		Skull crusher on stability ball with hip thrust	p. 146

(continued)

Table 11.2　Intermediate First Trimester Workout　*(continued)*

Activity	Program design		
Full-body strength training	**B**	Lateral raise	p. 152
		Seated march on stability ball	p. 88
		Crouching tiger	p. 98
		Side-lying triceps press-up	p. 145
		Side knee plank	p. 94
	C	Squat and back row	p. 123
		Straight-leg bridge with stability ball	p. 173
		Incline chest press on bench	p. 110
		Triceps press with stability ball	p. 142
		Bent-arm lateral raise	p. 156
		Seated march on stability ball	p. 88
		Crouching tiger	p. 98
		Side knee plank	p. 94
Functional movement	Functional movements are activities and movements that maintain or improve a person's ability to perform activities of daily living. Trying to incorporate these movements on a daily basis, or at least on most days, will help maintain the strength and endurance needed for labor, birth, and motherhood. *Walking:* Walk as much as you can, because it helps prepare you for labor and the many walks with the stroller, groceries, laundry, etc. *Climbing stairs:* If you live in a house or apartment with stairs, climbing stairs will help you better prepare for many trips up and down with baby, laundry, etc. *Squatting:* Along with deadlifts, these help strengthen the posterior chain and prepare for lifting loads. The squat and back row helps prepare for picking up the car seat and squatting to pick things up from the floor. *Lifting:* Performing deadlifts as part of your exercise program strengthens the posterior chain and helps prepare you for picking up the car seat and getting the baby in and out of the crib.		
Release work	Calf stretch		p. 67
	Hamstring stretch with strap		p. 71
	Feet on ball stretch		p. 66
	Seated chest stretch over stability ball		p. 63
	4 stretch		p. 70

ADVANCED

An advanced exerciser is someone who has extensive knowledge of fitness and exercise programming and who exercises four to five times per week at higher intensities. She is open to new challenges and likes to push herself to new heights. Barring complications, she will eagerly continue to exercise right through her pregnancy and will already have a plan in place for getting back into the gym after birth. See table 11.3 for a sample advanced first trimester workout.

Table 11.3 Advanced First Trimester Workout

Activity	Program design		
Cardio	If walking is your only cardio, then do it four to five days per week for at least 30 minutes per day on hilly terrain, or continue with your regular cardio regimen. We recommend a walk outside in nature or a hike every single day, even if you enjoy swimming or use a cardio machine.		
Full-body strength training	Do your strength training at least four days per week, performing three or more sets with 10 to 12 reps per set as tolerated. Choose one of the three workouts provided (A, B, or C) or, for a more individualized approach, choose exercises from each one and create your own workout (just make sure to hit all the major muscle groups—legs, chest, back, arms, core).		
	A	Squat on BOSU	p. 178
		Standing hamstring curl with stability ball	p. 166
		Straight-leg bridge with stability ball	p. 173
		Calf raise with stability ball	p. 161
		Walkover push-up on BOSU	p. 108
		One-leg deadlift	p. 182
		Preacher curl	p. 127
		Skull crusher on stability ball	p. 143
		Bent-arm lateral raise	p. 156
		Seated march on stability ball	p. 88
		Front loaded plank	p. 99
		Bird dog	p. 96
		Side knee plank	p. 94
		Cat and cow	p. 93
		Clam shell	p. 84

(continued)

Table 11.3   Advanced First Trimester Workout *(continued)*

Activity		Program design	
Full-body strength training	**B**	Squat on BOSU	p. 178
		Rear crescent lunge	p. 157
		Donkey kick	p. 167
		Calf raise with stability ball	p. 161
		Walkover push-up on BOSU	p. 108
		One-arm bent-over row	p. 118
		Skull crusher on stability ball with hip thrust	p. 146
		Seated march on stability ball	p. 88
		Pallof press	p. 100
		Bird dog	p. 96
		Side knee plank	p. 94
		Cat and cow	p. 93
		Clam shell	p. 84
	C	Squat on BOSU	p. 178
		Deadlift on BOSU	p. 180
		Stationary lunge with one foot on BOSU	p. 179
		Push-up	p. 112
		One-arm bent-over row	p. 118
		Ball squat with biceps curl	p. 139
		Seated triceps extension	p. 144
		Lateral raise	p. 152
		Seated march on stability ball	p. 88
		Front-loaded plank	p. 99
		Bird dog	p. 96
		Pallof press	p. 100
		Cat and cow	p. 93
		Side-lying bent knee lift	p. 85

Activity	Program design	
Functional movement	Functional movements are activities and movements that maintain or improve a person's ability to perform activities of daily living. Trying to incorporate these movements on a daily basis, or at least on most days, will help maintain the strength and endurance needed for labor, birth, and motherhood. *Walking:* Walk as much as you can, because it helps prepare you for labor and the many walks with the stroller, groceries, laundry, etc. *Climbing stairs:* If you live in a house or apartment with stairs, climbing stairs will help you better prepare for many trips up and down with baby, laundry, etc. *Lifting:* Performing deadlifts as part of your exercise program strengthens the posterior chain and helps prepare you for picking up the car seat and getting the baby in and out of the crib. *Squatting:* Along with deadlifts, these help strengthen the posterior chain and prepare for lifting loads. The squat on BOSU exercise helps you prepare for instability when squatting and lifting.	
Release work	Calf stretch	p. 67
	Hamstring stretch with strap	p. 71
	Feet on ball stretch	p. 66
	Seated chest stretch over stability ball	p. 63
	4 stretch	p. 70
	Rotate and reach stretch	p. 60

12

Second Trimester Workouts

Once you have entered your second trimester, energy levels begin to increase and nausea is usually a thing of the past. This is when the urge to get back to your routine returns for the intermediate and advanced exerciser and the beginner feels like she can perform a fitness routine comfortably and with confidence.

These next three months are when you are most likely to try a new exercise class or, if you are a regular exerciser, increase your intensity and push yourself a bit more. However, as "normal" as you may feel, you still have to remember all the changes that are happening and ensure you are being purposeful with your movement. Make your activities specific to labor preparation, modify your core work, and use caution with heavy lifting and high-impact activities.

You can still increase the intensity without adding impact. Hill walking, stair walking, stationary biking, and swimming are all great low-impact cardio activities. This is also a great time to train your balance and recruit your core before your center of gravity really starts to change.

One note of caution: some recommend that in your second and third trimesters you avoid lying on your back so you don't compress the vena cava. However, some women have no adverse effects from back-lying positions and may choose to continue exercising on their backs.

For exercises that are to be done in a supine (back lying) position, adjust your bench so you are on an incline or use a wedge or stack of pillows for supine floor work to keep your heart above your head. It is also important to pay attention to how you get into and out of incline or supine positions. When getting into the position, start on your side and then roll onto your back. When getting up, roll to your side and press your body back up to seated.

BEGINNER

A beginner exerciser is someone who has not been exercising or who exercises sporadically with little knowledge or expertise regarding fitness and exercise programming. She is uncertain about what exercises she can or cannot do and often feels intimidated about going to the gym. She struggles with maintaining a regular exercise routine and needs constant support and guidance. See table 12.1 for a sample beginner second trimester workout.

Table 12.1 Beginner Second Trimester Workout

Activity	Program design		
Cardio	Walk five days a week for 20 to 30 minutes per day. Your energy tends to increase and you feel more normal during the second trimester. You can also add other activities like swimming or Aquafit classes one to three days a week based on your fitness level.		
Full-body strength training	Do your strength training one to two days per week, performing two to three sets with 8 to 12 reps. Choose one of the three workouts provided (A, B, or C) or, for a more individualized approach, choose exercises from each one and create your own workout (just make sure to hit all the major muscle groups—legs, chest, back, arms, core).		
	A	Squat	p. 86
		Lunge	p. 90
		Seated hip adduction	p. 170
		Calf raise with stability ball	p. 161
		Incline chest press on bench	p. 110
		One-arm bent-over row	p. 118
		Barbell biceps curl	p. 132
		Triceps kickback	p. 141
		Lateral raise	p. 152
		Seated march on stability ball	p. 88
		Standing bird dog	p. 97
		Pelvic rocking on stability ball	p. 92
		Bridge	p. 83
	B	Squat and back row	p. 123
		Lunge with biceps curl	p. 136
		Stationary lunge with overhead triceps extension	p. 149

Activity		Program design	
Full-body strength training	**B**	Calf raise with stability ball	p. 161
		Wall push-up	p. 104
		Standing shoulder retraction	p. 116
		Seated lat pulldown	p. 117
		Seated march on stability ball	p. 88
		Standing bird dog	p. 97
		Pelvic rocking on stability ball	p. 92
		Clam shell	p. 84
	C	One-arm bent-over row	p. 118
		Deadlift	p. 172
		Calf raise with stability ball	p. 161
		Rear crescent lunge	p. 157
		Chest press with band	p. 106
		Bent-over reverse fly	p. 120
		Frankenstein walk	p. 176
		Core breath	p. 81
		Standing bird dog	p. 97
		Pelvic rocking on stability ball	p. 92
		Bridge	p. 83
Functional movement		Functional movements are activities and movements that maintain or improve a person's ability to perform activities of daily living. Trying to incorporate these movements on a daily basis, or at least on most days, will help maintain the strength and endurance needed for labor, birth, and motherhood. *Walking:* Walk as much as you can, because it helps prepare you for labor and the many walks with the stroller, groceries, laundry, etc. *Climbing stairs:* If you live in a house or apartment with stairs, climbing stairs will help you better prepare for many trips up and down with baby, laundry, etc. *Squatting:* Along with deadlifts, these help strengthen the posterior chain and prepare for lifting loads. *Lifting:* Performing deadlifts as part of your exercise program strengthens the posterior chain and helps prepare you for picking up the car seat and getting the baby in and out of the crib. *Lunges:* These help strengthen your legs for both walking and stairs. The rear crescent lunge helps prepare you for balance and reaching into the back seat for baby.	

(continued)

Table 12.1 Beginner Second Trimester Workout *(continued)*

Activity	Program design	
Release work	Calf stretch	p. 67
	Hamstring stretch with strap	p. 71
	Seated chest stretch over stability ball	p. 63
	Side-lying stretch over ball	p. 64
	Psoas release with bolster	p. 72
	4 stretch	p. 70
	Pelvic rocking on stability ball	p. 92

INTERMEDIATE

An intermediate exerciser is someone who regularly exercises two to three times per week with a good understanding of fitness for health and weight management. She feels confident in the gym and tries a variety of different exercise routines and techniques. She enjoys fitness and understands it's a part of her lifestyle. See table 12.2 for a sample intermediate second trimester workout.

Table 12.2 Intermediate Second Trimester Workout

Activity	Program design		
Cardio	If walking is your only cardio, then do it four to five days per week for at least 30 minutes per day on hilly terrain, or continue with your regular cardio regimen. We recommend a walk outside in nature or a hike every single day, even if you enjoy swimming or use a cardio machine. Aim for some form of cardio (such as hiking, swimming, Aquafit classes, or gym activities) and a walk four to five days per week.		
Full-body strength training	Do your strength training two to three days per week, using both free weights and your body weight. Only increase the amount of weight being lifted if you can perform two to three sets of 10 to 12 reps comfortably. Choose one of the three workouts provided (A, B, or C) or, for a more individualized approach, choose exercises from each one and create your own workout (just make sure to hit all the major muscle groups—legs, chest, back, arms, core).		
	A	Hip thrust	p. 181
		Deadlift and back row	p. 174
		Walking lunge	p. 171
		Calf raise with stability ball	p. 161
		Wall push-up	p. 104
		Bent-over reverse fly	p. 120
		Hammer curl and shoulder press	p. 134
		Skull crusher	p. 140
		Seated march on stability ball	p. 88
		Ball squeeze rotation	p. 95
		Pallof press	p. 100
	B	Monster walk	p. 184
		Lunge with biceps curl	p. 136
		Frankenstein walk	p. 176

(continued)

Table 12.2   Intermediate Second Trimester Workout *(continued)*

Activity		Program design	
Full-body strength training	**B**	Wall push-up	p. 104
		Bent-over reverse fly	p. 120
		Preacher curl	p. 127
		Side-lying triceps press-up	p. 145
		Seated march on stability ball	p. 88
		Ball squeeze rotation	p. 95
		Kneeling ball squeeze	p. 109
	C	Car seat squat	p. 188
		Deadlift and back row	p. 174
		Calf raise with stability ball	p. 161
		Incline chest press on bench	p. 110
		Bent-over reverse fly	p. 120
		One-leg deadlift	p. 182
		Triceps press with stability ball	p. 142
		Alternating front raise	p. 155
		Pallof press	p. 100
		Standing bird dog	p. 97
		One-arm reverse fly	p. 114
		Crab walk	p. 147
Functional movement		Functional movements are activities and movements that maintain or improve a person's ability to perform activities of daily living. Trying to incorporate these movements on a daily basis, or at least on most days, will help maintain the strength and endurance needed for labor, birth, and motherhood. *Walking:* Walk as much as you can, because it helps prepare you for labor and the many walks with the stroller, groceries, laundry, etc. *Climbing stairs:* If you live in a house or apartment with stairs, climbing stairs will help you better prepare for many trips up and down with baby, laundry, etc. *Lifting:* Performing deadlifts as part of your exercise program strengthens the posterior chain and helps prepare you for picking up the car seat and getting the baby in and out of the crib. *Squatting:* Along with deadlifts, these help strengthen the posterior chain and prepare for lifting loads.	

Activity	Program design	
Release work	Calf stretch	p. 67
	Hamstring stretch with strap	p. 61
	Seated chest stretch over stability ball	p. 63
	Side-lying stretch over ball	p. 64
	Psoas release with bolster	p. 72
	4 stretch	p. 70
	Rotate and reach stretch	p. 60

ADVANCED

An advanced exerciser is someone who has extensive knowledge of fitness and exercise programming and who exercises four to five times per week at higher intensities. She is open to new challenges and likes to push herself to new heights. Barring complications, she will eagerly continue to exercise right through her pregnancy and will already have a plan in place for getting back into the gym after birth. See table 12.3 for a sample advanced second trimester workout.

Table 12.3 Advanced Second Trimester Workout

Activity	Program design		
Cardio	Walk five days per week for 30 or more minutes per day. You may also want to try hill walking, the elliptical machine, or a stationary bike. We recommend a walk outside in nature or a hike every single day, even if you enjoy swimming or use a cardio machine.		
Full-body strength training	Do your strength training three to four days per week. Only increase the amount of weight being lifted if you can perform three or more sets of 8 to 12 reps comfortably. Choose one of the three workouts provided (A, B, or C) or, for a more individualized approach, choose exercises from each one and create your own workout (just make sure to hit all the major muscle groups—legs, chest, back, arms, core).		
	A	Car seat squat	p. 188
		Deadlift	p. 172
		Squat and back row	p. 123
		Calf raise with stability ball	p. 161
		Wall push-up	p. 104
		Standing upright row with band	p. 151
		Standing hammer curl	p. 131
		Triceps press with stability ball	p. 142
		One-arm reverse fly	p. 114
		Seated march on stability ball	p. 88
		Pallof press	p. 100
		Standing bird dog	p. 97
		Side knee plank	p. 94
		Straight-leg bridge with stability ball	p. 173
		Clam shell	p. 84

Activity		Program design	
Full-body strength training	**B**	Stationary lunge with one foot on BOSU	p. 179
		Monster walk	p. 184
		Preacher curl	p. 127
		One-leg deadlift	p. 182
		Squat and back row	p. 123
		Skull crusher on stability ball with hip thrust	p. 146
		Seated shoulder press	p. 154
		Kneeling ball squeeze	p. 109
		Standing bird dog	p. 97
		Side knee plank	p. 94
		Side-lying bent knee lift	p. 85
	C	Frankenstein walk	p. 176
		Lunge and one-arm row	p. 125
		Deadlift	p. 172
		Side-lying triceps press-up	p. 145
		Bent-arm lateral raise	p. 156
		Bent-over reverse fly	p. 120
		Alternating front raise	p. 155
		Standing bird dog	p. 97
		Side knee plank	p. 94
		Core breath	p. 81

(continued)

Table 12.3   Advanced Second Trimester Workout *(continued)*

Activity	Program design	
Functional movement	Functional movements are activities and movements that maintain or improve a person's ability to perform activities of daily living. Trying to incorporate these movements on a daily basis, or at least on most days, will help maintain the strength and endurance needed for labor, birth, and motherhood. *Walking:* Walk as much as you can, because it helps prepare you for labor and the many walks with the stroller, groceries, laundry, etc. *Climbing stairs:* If you live in a house or apartment with stairs, climbing stairs will help you better prepare for many trips up and down with baby, laundry, etc. *Lifting:* Performing deadlifts as part of your exercise program strengthens the posterior chain and helps prepare you for picking up the car seat and getting the baby in and out of the crib. The deadlift and back row is especially helpful for this. *Squatting:* Along with deadlifts, these help strengthen the posterior chain and prepare for lifting loads. The car seat squat helps prepare you for the instability and balance challenge of carrying a car seat.	
Release work	Calf stretch	p. 67
	Hamstring stretch with strap	p. 71
	4 stretch	p. 70
	Seated chest stretch over stability ball	p. 63

Third Trimester Workouts

13

The third trimester is when most women will naturally begin to scale back their exercise routine, whether it's reducing the number of sets, repetitions, or the amount of weight being lifted. During this time, you are gaining between a half to one pound (0.25 to 0.5 kg) each week and may be suffering from varicose veins, increased fluid retention, swelling, and overall difficulty carrying around the extra weight load. The Core 4 muscles are becoming overstretched and their normal function is becoming more and more compromised as they try to manage the increased load.

As baby and the uterus continue to grow, they increase demands on the body, which can lower your energy levels. As with any physically demanding event, the goal should be to try to maintain consistency with your exercise routine, doing at least some work most days of the week. Whether it's in the weight room, outdoors, or in a swimming pool, maintaining the routine of being physically active is key.

The third trimester is also when you'll increase your focus on preparing for the big event. Add specific exercises that will help you in labor and birth to your routine. Deep squats, stretch and release work, and breathing techniques for birth will round out your programming.

BEGINNER

A beginner exerciser is someone who has not been exercising or who exercises sporadically with little knowledge or expertise regarding fitness and exercise programming. She is uncertain about what exercises she can or cannot do and often feels intimidated about going to the gym. She struggles with maintaining a regular exercise routine and needs constant support and guidance. See table 13.1 for a sample beginner third trimester workout.

Table 13.1 Beginner Third Trimester Workout

Activity	Program design		
Cardio	It's normal to cut back at some point during this trimester. Stop exercising once you feel tired (don't work to exhaustion). Walk three to five days a week, 20 to 30 minutes per day. You can also continue to swim if it feels good. Low-intensity Aquafit classes are a good option too. The buoyancy of the water feels especially good during the later stages of pregnancy.		
Full-body strength training	Do strength training as tolerated, one to two days per week, using both free weights and your body weight., Do one to two sets of 8 to 12 reps. Choose one of the three workouts provided (A, B, or C) or, for a more individualized approach, choose exercises from each one and create your own workout (just make sure to hit all the major muscle groups—legs, chest, back, arms, core).		
	A	Stability ball squat	p. 162
		Standing hip abduction with ball	p. 168
		Wall push-up	p. 104
		Seated back row	p. 115
		Seated biceps curl	p. 133
		Seated triceps extension	p. 144
		Standing lat pulldown	p. 124
		Ball squeeze rotation	p. 95
		Seated hip adduction	p. 170
		Bridge	p. 83
		Core breath (modified)	p. 81
	B	Stability ball lunge	p. 164
		Standing hamstring curl with stability ball	p. 166
		Calf raise with stability ball	p. 161
		Incline chest press on bench	p. 110

Activity	Program design		
Full-body strength training	**B**	Bent-over reverse fly	p. 120
		Triceps kickback	p. 141
		Upright row	p. 121
		Ball squeeze rotation	p. 95
		Seated hip abduction	p. 169
		Core breath (modified)	p. 81
	C	Stability ball lunge	p. 164
		Standing hamstring curl with stability ball	p. 166
		Calf raise with stability ball	p. 161
		Wall push-up	p. 104
		One-arm bent-over row	p. 118
		Skull crusher	p. 140
		Standing shoulder retraction	p. 116
		Seated march on stability ball	p. 88
		Core breath (modified)	p. 81
		Bridge	p. 83
		Clam shell	p. 84
Functional movement	Functional movements are activities and movements that maintain or improve a person's ability to perform activities of daily living. Trying to incorporate these movements on a daily basis, or at least on most days, will help maintain the strength and endurance needed for labor, birth, and motherhood. *Walking:* Walk as much as you can, because it helps prepare you for labor and the many walks with the stroller, groceries, laundry, etc. *Climbing stairs:* If you live in a house or apartment with stairs, climbing stairs will help you better prepare for many trips up and down with baby, laundry, etc. *Squatting:* Along with deadlifts, these help strengthen the posterior chain and prepare for lifting loads. *Lifting:* Performing deadlifts as part of your exercise program strengthens the posterior chain and helps prepare you for picking up the car seat and getting the baby in and out of the crib.		

(continued)

Table 13.1   Beginner Third Trimester Workout *(continued)*

Activity	Program design	
Release work	Calf stretch	p. 67
	Hamstring stretch with strap	p. 71
	Seated chest stretch over stability ball	p. 63
	Side-lying stretch over ball	p. 64
	Psoas release with bolster	p. 72
	Posterior pelvic floor release	p. 74
	Pelvic rocking on stability ball	p. 92
	Adductor stretch on stability ball	p. 68
	Hip flexor stretch on stability ball	p. 69
	4 stretch	p. 70

INTERMEDIATE

An intermediate exerciser is someone who regularly exercises two to three times per week with a good understanding of fitness for health and weight management. She feels confident in the gym and tries a variety of different exercise routines and techniques. She enjoys fitness and understands it's a part of her lifestyle. See table 13.2 for a sample intermediate third trimester workout.

Table 13.2 Intermediate Third Trimester Workout

Activity	Program design		
Cardio	It's normal to cut back at some point during this trimester. Stop exercising once you feel tired (don't work to exhaustion). Walk three to five days a week, 20 to 30 minutes per day. You can also continue to swim if it feels good. Low-intensity Aquafit classes are a good option too. The buoyancy of the water feels especially good during the later stages of pregnancy.		
Full-body strength training	Do your strength training two to three days per week, with two to three sets of 10 to 12 reps or what you can comfortably complete. Listen to your body and adjust the amount of weight as needed. Place more focus on preparing for birth. Choose one of the three workouts provided (A, B, or C) or, for a more individualized approach, choose exercises from each one and create your own workout (just make sure to hit all the major muscle groups—legs, chest, back, arms, core).		
	A	Car seat squat	p. 188
		Deadlift and back row	p. 174
		Calf raise with stability ball	p. 161
		Kneeling ball squeeze	p. 109
		Standing lat pulldown	p. 124
		Standing hammer curl	p. 131
		Triceps kickback	p. 141
		Lateral raise	p. 152
		Seated march on stability ball	p. 88
		Standing bird dog	p. 97
		Ball squeeze rotation	p. 95
		Bridge	p. 83
		Core breath (modified)	p. 81

(continued)

Table 13.2   Intermediate Third Trimester Workout *(continued)*

Activity		Program design	
Full-body strength training	**B**	Squat and back row	p. 123
		Rear crescent lunge	p. 157
		Calf raise with stability ball	p. 161
		Chest press with band	p. 106
		One-arm reverse fly	p. 114
		Triceps press with stability ball	p. 142
		Seated march on stability ball	p. 88
		Standing bird dog	p. 97
		Kneeling hover	p. 183
		Side-lying bent knee lift	p. 85
		Pallof press	p. 100
		Core breath (modified)	p. 81
	C	Squat	p. 86
		Standing hip abduction with ball	p. 168
		Upright row	p. 121
		Barbell biceps curl	p. 132
		Standing shoulder retraction	p. 116
		Seated march on stability ball	p. 88
		Standing bird dog	p. 97
		Lateral raise	p. 152
		Bridge	p. 83
		Side knee plank	p. 94
		Side-lying bent-knee lift	p. 85
		Core breath (modified)	p. 81

Activity	Program design	
Functional movement	Functional movements are activities and movements that maintain or improve a person's ability to perform activities of daily living. Trying to incorporate these movements on a daily basis, or at least on most days, will help maintain the strength and endurance needed for labor, birth, and motherhood. *Walking:* Walk as much as you can, because it helps prepare you for labor and the many walks with the stroller, groceries, laundry, etc. *Climbing stairs:* If you live in a house or apartment with stairs, climbing stairs will help you better prepare for many trips up and down with baby, laundry, etc. *Squatting:* Along with deadlifts, these help strengthen the posterior chain and prepare for lifting loads. The car seat squat especially helps prepare you for the instability of carrying a heavy load on one side. *Lifting:* Performing deadlifts as part of your exercise program strengthens the posterior chain and helps prepare you for picking up the car seat and getting the baby in and out of the crib.	
Release work	Calf stretch	p. 67
	Hamstring stretch with strap	p. 71
	Seated chest stretch over stability ball	p. 63
	Side-lying stretch over ball	p. 64
	Psoas release with bolster	p. 72
	Posterior pelvic floor release with ball	p. 74
	Pelvic rocking on stability ball	p. 92
	Hip flexor stretch on stability ball	p. 69
	4 stretch	p. 70
	Adductor stretch on stability ball	p. 68

ADVANCED

An advanced exerciser is someone who has extensive knowledge of fitness and exercise programming and who exercises four to five times per week at higher intensities. She is open to new challenges and likes to push herself to new heights. Barring complications, she will eagerly continue to exercise right through her pregnancy and will already have a plan in place for getting back into the gym after birth. See table 13.3 for a sample advanced third trimester workout.

Table 13.3 Advanced Third Trimester Workout

Activity	Program design		
Cardio	It's normal to cut back at some point during this trimester. Stop exercising once you feel tired (don't work to exhaustion). Walk five days per week for 30 minutes per day. Adjust intensity and speed as needed. Continue with hills as tolerated. You can also continue to swim or participate in low-intensity Aquafit classes if it feels good. The buoyancy of the water feels especially good during the later stages of pregnancy.		
Full-body strength training	Do your strength training three to four days per week, using both free weights and your body weight. Decrease the amount of weight lifted as needed. Complete three sets of 8 to 12 repetitions. Choose one of the three workouts provided (A, B, or C) or, for a more individualized approach, choose exercises from each one and create your own workout (just make sure to hit all the major muscle groups—legs, chest, back, arms, core).		
	A	Squat and back row	p. 123
		Deadlift	p. 172
		Calf raise with stability ball	p. 161
		Incline chest press on bench	p. 110
		Ball squat with biceps curl	p. 139
		Skull crusher on stability ball	p. 143
		Lateral raise	p. 152
		Seated march on stability ball	p. 88
		Ball squeeze rotation	p. 95
		Standing bird dog	p. 97
		Kneeling hover	p. 183
		Clam shell	p. 84
		Bridge	p. 83

Activity		Program design	
Full-body strength training	**B**	Lunge with biceps curl	p. 136
		Stationary lunge with overhead triceps extension	p. 149
		Squat and back row	p. 123
		Preacher curl	p. 127
		Triceps press with stability ball	p. 142
		Seated shoulder press	p. 154
		Seated march on stability ball	p. 88
		Pallof press	p. 100
		Standing bird dog	p. 97
		One-arm reverse fly	p. 114
		Side-lying bent-knee lift	p. 85
		Bridge	p. 83
	C	Ball squat with biceps curl	p. 139
		Frankenstein walk	p. 176
		Deadlift and back row	p. 174
		Calf raise with stability ball	p. 161
		Standing upright row with band	p. 151
		Hammer curl and shoulder press	p. 134
		Hip thrust	p. 181
		Seated march on stability ball	p. 88
		Standing bird dog	p. 97
		Standing shoulder retraction	p. 116
		Clam shell	p. 84
		Bridge	p. 83

(continued)

Table 13.3 Advanced Third Trimester Workout *(continued)*

Activity	Program design	
Functional movement	Functional movements are activities and movements that maintain or improve a person's ability to perform activities of daily living. Trying to incorporate these movements on a daily basis, or at least on most days, will help maintain the strength and endurance needed for labor, birth, and motherhood. *Walking:* Walk as much as you can, because it helps prepare you for labor and the many walks with the stroller, groceries, laundry, etc. *Climbing stairs:* If you live in a house or apartment with stairs, climbing stairs will help you better prepare for many trips up and down with baby, laundry, etc. *Lifting:* Performing deadlifts as part of your exercise program strengthens the posterior chain and helps prepare you for picking up the car seat and getting the baby in and out of the crib. *Squatting:* Along with deadlifts, these help strengthen the posterior chain and prepare for lifting loads. The squat and shoulder press especially helps you prepare for deep squatting and lifting your baby	
Release work	Calf stretch	p. 67
	Hamstring stretch with strap	p. 71
	Seated chest stretch over stability ball	p. 63
	Side-lying stretch over ball	p. 64
	Psoas release with bolster	p. 72
	Posterior pelvic floor release	p. 74
	Pelvic rocking on stability ball	p. 92
	Hip flexor stretch on stability ball	p. 69
	Adductor stretch on stability ball	p. 68
	4 stretch	p. 70

14

Fourth Trimester Workouts

The moment your baby is born, you are filled with the most incredible feelings in the world. You are then officially a mom and have entered the postpartum recovery phase. The first eight weeks are the most important when it comes to healing the body and restoring your core and abdominal wall. The exercises listed in this chapter can help anyone who wants to retrain their inner core and get back to her desired activities, even if you are reading this after the first eight weeks postpartum. The key is to remember that recovery is essential and that the core needs to be retrained before it can be trained. The Core 4 have undergone a lot of stretch and strain, and the synergy needs to be regained before the body resumes regular physical activity. If you go too hard too soon, you may be setting yourself up for some challenges down the road. Take the time now to rest, recover and retrain. You will be glad you did!

Pregnancy and birth are physically, emotionally, and mentally taxing, so when you resume your exercise routine during recovery, it is important to go back to basics. This may make sense to the beginner exerciser but may be a challenge for the intermediate and advanced exerciser. Most women are excited about the prospect of not being pregnant anymore, of getting their body back and of feeling like themselves again. New moms are drawn to activities such as boot camp and high-intensity interval activities because they think that will help them feel strong again and get them there quickly. However, we urge you to take it slow, rebuild your inner core, and progress back gradually to these activities. We are not saying you can never do boot camp again. We are saying that boot camp should not be what you use to get your body back.

Like with any major physical event, remember that rest and recovery are of utmost importance in ensuring that you can go back to your desired activities without injury. Everyone will progress at a different rate, so be true to yourself, take your time, and allow your body to recover. Also, keep in mind that your new baby may keep you from getting a good night's sleep, and if you haven't slept well your tolerance for exercise will be less. On days when you have had little sleep, do less but do something, even if you have to bring it down a notch or two compared to yesterday or last week. It will all come back when you do it right.

Once you begin to build up your function, strength, and stamina, you can start to be creative with your exercise. You don't have to be stuck in a gym or exercise class (although those can be a nice escape when they offer child care). Use your daily walks (now with a stroller or carrier) as your workout. The added weight of the stroller acts as resistance and will amp up your cardio. You can use park benches and playground equipment to assist your squats and some stretches. Swimming is a fantastic cardiovascular workout and water aerobics have come a long way with intensity and strength-building. Hiking, cycling, spinning, and low-impact exercise classes are great alternatives to keep you motivated in your fitness goals. But even though these are all good choices beyond the first eight weeks, remember to wait until you have had time to rest and heal and you have had your first pelvic floor physiotherapy assessment. Go slow; it's not a race.

The following exercise programs give you a variety of choices you need in the gym or in your home to focus on your core and slowly rebuild while ensuring safety and support.

RECOVER AND RETRAIN

Starting a program after birth can be challenging. You'll be facing a demanding newborn, sleep deprivation, and a body that needs to recover, so start slow and build as you feel comfortable.

This workout is for all fitness levels during the first eight weeks after birth. Whether you are a beginner, an intermediate, or an advanced exerciser or athlete, everyone must start at the beginning in order to rebuild a strong foundation. See table 14.1 for a sample recover and retrain workout.

Start with the core breath once a day for three to five minutes. A good time might be after you put your baby down for a nap or while feeding. Each week, add one exercise as tolerated. Do as many reps as you can with perfect form once a day (most days of the week), but don't put too much pressure on yourself, because one day can be very different from the other.

Try to carve out time to do your exercises when you have the most energy and can focus (usually in the morning). Remember to practice perfection instead of trying to do a certain number of sets or reps. If you can do eight perfectly but fail at nine, stop and start again the next day.

RESTORE

Once you have completed the eight-week retraining exercises, you are feeling good, and you have been assessed by a pelvic floor physiotherapist, it is time to gently increase the intensity so you can progress from what you

Table 14.1 Sample Recover and Retrain Workout

Week 1	Core breath (side-lying or supine until your perineum has healed)	p. 81
Week 2	Core breath	p. 81
	Bridge	p. 83
Week 3	Core breath	p. 81
	Bridge	p. 83
	Clam shell	p. 84
Week 4	Core breath	p. 81
	Bridge	p. 83
	Clam shell	p. 84
	Side-lying bent-knee lift	p. 85
Week 5	Core breath	p. 81
	Bridge	p. 83
	Clam shell	p. 84
	Side-lying bent-knee lift	p. 85
	Seated march on stability ball	p. 88
Week 6	Core breath	p. 81
	Bridge	p. 83
	Clam shell	p. 84
	Side-lying bent-knee lift	p. 85
	Seated march on stability ball	p. 88
	Stability ball squat	p. 162
Week 7	Core breath	p. 81
	Bridge	p. 83
	Clam shell	p. 84
	Side-lying bent-knee lift	p. 85
	Seated march on stability ball	p. 88
	Squat	p. 86
	Standing one-leg transfer	p. 89
Week 8	Core breath	p. 81
	Bridge	p. 83
	Clam shell	p. 84
	Side-lying bent-knee lift	p. 85
	Seated march on stability ball	p. 88
	Squat	p. 86
	Standing one-leg transfer	p. 89
	Stability ball lunge	p. 164

have already built. The following exercise programs give you a good variety of safe and functional exercises that continue to focus on core stability while improving posture, strength, and mobility.

You will want to continue doing the core breath daily, but the exercise routines can be completed one to four times per week (depending on fitness level) with one to three sets of 6 to 12 repetitions. Start with workout A in the first week, then try B the following week, and so on. However, feel free to also pick out some of your favorite exercises and create your own workout.

Beginner

A beginner exerciser is someone who has not been exercising or who exercises sporadically with little knowledge or expertise regarding fitness and exercise programming. She is uncertain about what exercises she can or cannot do and often feels intimidated about going to the gym. She struggles with maintaining a regular exercise routine and needs constant support and guidance. See table 14.2 for a sample beginner workout to restore.

Table 14.2 Sample Beginner Restore Workout

Activity	Program design		
Cardio	Do gentle walking starting with 5 to 10 minutes per day, adding two to three minutes each week.		
Full-body strength training	Do your strength training one to two days per week, doing one to two sets of six to eight reps. All seated positions can be performed on a chair or stability ball.		
	A	Squat	p. 86
		Seated lat pulldown	p. 117
		Seated biceps curl	p. 133
		Seated triceps extension	p. 144
		Standing upright row with band	p. 151
		Seated hip abduction	p. 169
		Bridge	p. 83
		Side-lying bent-knee lift	p. 85

Activity		Program design	
Full-body strength training	**B**	Frankenstein walk	p. 176
		Lunge	p. 90
		Standing hammer curl	p. 131
		Skull crusher	p. 140
		Standing upright row with band	p. 151
		Seated march on stability ball	p. 88
		Kneeling hover	p. 183
		Side-lying bent-knee lift	p. 85
	C	Lunge	p. 90
		Standing one-arm back row	p. 122
		Preacher curl	p. 127
		Triceps kickback	p. 141
		Standing shoulder retraction	p. 116
		Seated march on stability ball	p. 88
		Bridge	p. 83
		Side-lying bent-knee lift	p. 85
Release work		Calf stretch	p. 67
		Hamstrings stretch with strap	p. 71
		Seated chest stretch over stability ball	p. 63
		Psoas release with bolster	p. 72
		Rotate and reach stretch	p. 60
		4 stretch	p. 70

Intermediate

An intermediate exerciser is someone who regularly exercises two to three times per week with a good understanding of fitness for health and weight management. She feels confident in the gym and tries a variety of different exercise routines and techniques. She enjoys fitness and understands it's a part of her lifestyle. See table 14.3 for a sample intermediate workout to restore.

Table 14.3 Sample Intermediate Restore Workout

Activity	Program design		
Cardio	Do gentle walking starting with 5 to 10 minutes per day, adding two to three minutes each week.		
Full-body strength training	Do your strength training one to two days per week, using free weights and your body weight, doing one to two sets of six to eight reps. All seated positions can be performed on a chair or stability ball.		
	A	Car seat squat	p. 188
		Lunge	p. 90
		Kneeling ball squeeze	p. 109
		Standing lat pulldown	p. 124
		Seated biceps curl	p. 133
		Skull crusher on stability ball	p. 143
		Seated hip abduction	p. 169
		Seated march on stability ball	p. 88
		Standing bird dog	p. 97
	B	Standing hip abduction with ball	p. 168
		Rear crescent lunge	p. 157
		Wall push-up	p. 104
		One-arm reverse fly	p. 114
		Incline biceps curl on bench	p. 130
		Skull crusher	p. 140

Activity	Program design		
Full-body strength training	**B**	Upright row	p. 121
		Seated hip adduction	p. 170
		Seated march on stability ball	p. 88
		Standing bird dog	p. 97
		Pallof press	p. 100
		Side knee plank	p. 94
	C	Laundry squat	p. 209
		Monster walk	p. 184
		Incline chest press (use variation on the floor)	p. 110
		Standing one-arm back row	p. 122
		Standing hammer curl	p. 131
		Seated triceps extension	p. 144
		Bent-arm lateral raise	p. 156
		Seated hip abduction	p. 169
		Seated march on stability ball	p. 88
		Standing bird dog	p. 97
		Bridge	p. 83
		Clam shell	p. 84
		Side-lying bent-knee lift	p. 85
Release work	Calf stretch		p. 67
	Hamstrings stretch with strap		p. 71
	Seated chest stretch over stability ball		p. 63
	Standing C-stretch		p. 62
	4 stretch		p. 70
	Psoas release with bolster		p. 72

Advanced

An advanced exerciser is someone who has extensive knowledge of fitness and exercise programming and who exercises four to five times per week at higher intensities. She is open to new challenges and likes to push herself to new heights. Barring complications, she will eagerly continue to exercise right through her pregnancy and will already have a plan in place for getting back into the gym after birth. See table 14.4 for a sample advanced workout to restore.

Table 14.4 Sample Advanced Restore Workout

Activity	Program design		
Cardio	Do gentle walking starting with 5 to 10 minutes per day, adding three to five minutes each week.		
Full-body strength training	Do your strength training two to four days per week, using free weights and your body weight, doing one to two sets of 8 to 10 reps. All seated positions can be performed on a chair or stability ball.		
	A	Squat and back row	p. 123
		Deadlift	p. 172
		Bridge	p. 83
		Push-up	p. 112
		Concentration curl	p. 138
		Triceps kickback	p. 141
		Standing upright row with band	p. 151
		Seated hip abduction	p. 169
		Seated march on stability ball	p. 88
		Standing bird dog	p. 97
		Crab walk	p. 147
		Clam shell	p. 84
		Side-lying bent-knee lift	p. 85
	B	Lunge	p. 90
		Ball squat with biceps curl	p. 139
		Skull crusher on stability ball with hip thrust	p. 146
		Incline chest press on bench	p. 110
		Standing shoulder retraction	p. 116

Activity	Program design			
Full-body strength training	**B**	Monster walk	p. 184
		Seated triceps extension	p. 144
		Seated hip abduction	p. 169
		Seated march on stability ball	p. 88
		Bird dog	p. 96
		Crouching tiger	p. 98
		Clam shell	p. 84
		Side-lying bent-knee lift	p. 85
	C	Squat	p. 86
		Deadlift and back row	p. 174
		Monster walk	p. 184
		Chest press with band	p. 106
		Hammer curl and shoulder press	p. 134
		Triceps press with stability ball	p. 142
		Bent-over reverse fly	p. 120
		Seated hip abduction	p. 169
		Seated march on stability ball	p. 88
		Standing bird dog	p. 97
		Standing biceps curl on BOSU	p. 137
		Bridge	p. 83
		Clam shell	p. 84
		Side-lying bent-knee lift	p. 85
Release work		Calf stretch	p. 67
		Hamstrings stretch with strap	p. 71
		Seated chest stretch over stability ball	p. 63
		Standing C-stretch	p. 62
		4 stretch	p. 70
		Psoas release with bolster	p. 72

BIBLIOGRAPHY

American Congress of Obstetricians and Gynecologists. 2017. "Frequently Asked Questions: Exercise During Pregnancy." July 2017. www.acog.org/Patients/FAQs/Exercise-During-Pregnancy.

American Congress of Obstetricians and Gynecologists Committee on Obstetric Practice. 2015. "Committee Opinion: Physical Activity and Exercise During Pregnancy and the Postpartum Period." December 2015 (reaffirmed 2017).

Austin, K., and B. Seebohar. 2011. *Performance Nutrition: Applying the Science of Nutrient Timing*. Champaign, IL: Human Kinetics.

Axer, H., D.G. Keyserlingk, and A. Prescher. 2001. "Collagen Fibers in Linea Alba and Rectus Sheaths II: Variability and Biomechanical Aspects." *Journal of Surgical Research* 96 (2): 239-45.

Beer, G. M., A. Schuster, B. Seifert, M. Manestar, D. Mihic-Probst, and S.A. Weber. 2009. "The Normal Width of the Linea Alba in Nulliparous Women." *Clinical Anatomy* 22:706-11.

Bø, K., and G. Hilde. 2013. "Does It Work in the Long Term? A Systematic Review on Pelvic Floor Muscle Training for Female Stress Urinary Incontinence." *Neurourology and Urodynamics* 32 (3): 215-23.

Bø, K., S. Mørkved, H. Frawley, and M. Sherburn. 2009. "Evidence for Benefit of Transversus Abdominis Training Alone or in Combination With Pelvic Floor Muscle Training to Treat Female Urinary Incontinence: A Systematic Review." *Neurourology and Urodynamics* 28 (5): 368-73.

Boissonnault, J.S., and M.J. Blaschak. 1988. "Incidence of Diastasis Recti Abdominis During Childbearing Year." *Physical Therapy* 68 (7): 1082-86.

Boissonnault, J.S., and R.K. Kotarinos. 1988. "Diastasis Recti I." In *Obstetric and Gynecologic Physical Therapy*, edited by E. Wilder, 63-81. New York: Churchill Livingstone.

Brauman, D. 2008. "Diastasis Recti: Clinical Anatomy." *Plastic and Reconstructive Surgery* 122 (5): 1564-9.

Brown, H.L. 2016. "Physiology of Pregnancy." Merck Manual. October 2016. www.merckmanuals.com/professional/gynecology-and-obstetrics/approach-to-the-pregnant-woman-and-prenatal-care/physiology-of-pregnancy.

Bruusgaard, J.C., I.B. Johansen, I.M. Engner, Z.A. Rana, and K. Gundersen. 2010. "Myonuclei Acquired by Overload Exercise Precede Hypertrophy and Are Not Lost on Detraining." *Proceedings of the National Academy of Sciences of the United States of America* 107, 15111-6. www.pnas.org/content/107/34/15111.full.pdf.

Cheifetz, O., S.D. Lucy, T.J. Overend, and J. Crowe. 2010. "The Effect of Abdominal Support on Functional Outcomes in Patients Following Major Abdominal Surgery: A Randomized Controlled Trial." *Physiotherapy Canada* 62 (3): 242-53. www.ncbi.nlm.nih.gov/pmc/articles/PMC2909864.

Chiarello, C.M., L.A. Falzone, K.E. McCaslin, M.N. Patel, and K.R. Ulery. 2005. "The Effects of an Exercise Program on Diastasis Recti Abdominis in Pregnant Women." *Journal of Women's Health Physical Therapy* 29 (1): 11-16.

Chiarello, C.M., and A. McAuley. 2014. "Mind the Gap: A Comprehensive Approach for the Evaluation of and Intervention of Diastasis Recti Abdominis." Las Vegas, NV: APTA Section on Women's Health.

Coldron, Y., M.J. Stokes, D.J. Newham, and K. Cook. 2008. "Postpartum Characteristics of Rectus Abdominis on Ultrasound Imaging." *Manual Therapy* 13:112-21.

da Mota, P.G., A.G. Pascoal, A. Carita, and K. Bø. 2014. "Prevalance and Risk Factors of Diastasis Recti Abdominis From Late Pregnancy to 6 Months Postpartum, and Relationship With Lumbo-Pelvic Pain." *Manual Therapy* 20 (1): 200-205. https://doi.org/10.1016/j.math.2014.09.002.

Davenport, M.H., S. Charlesworth, D. Vanderspank, M.M. Sopper, and M.F. Mottola, 2008. "Development and Validation of Exercise Target Heart Rate Zones for Overweight and Obese Pregnant Women," *Applied Physiology, Nutrition, and Metabolism* 33(5): 984-989.

Davies, G.A., L.A. Wolfe, M.F. Mottola, C. MacKinnon, M.Y. Arsenault, E. Bartellas, Y. Cargill, et al. 2003. "Exercise in Pregnancy and the Postpartum Period." *Journal of Obstetrics and Gynaecology Canada* 25 (6): 516-22.

Dempsey, F.C., Butler, F.L., and Williams, F.A. et al. 2005. "No Need for a Pregnant Pause: Physical Activity May Reduce the Occurrence of Gestational Diabetes Mellitus and Preeclampsia." Exercise and Sport Sciences Reviews 33(3): 141-149.

Dumoulin, C., and J. Hay-Smith. 2010. "Pelvic Floor Muscle Training Versus No Treatment, or Inactive Control Treatments, for Urinary Incontinence in Women." Cochrane Database of Systematic Reviews.

Eliasson, K., B. Elfving, B. Nordgren, and E. Mattsson. 2008. "Urinary Incontinence in Women With Low Back Pain." *Manual Therapy* 13:206-12.

Field, T., Figueiredo, B., Hernandez-Reif, M., Diego, M., Deeds, O., and Ascencio, A. 2008. "Massage Therapy Reduces Pain in Pregnant Women, Alleviates Prenatal Depression in Both Parents and Improves Their Relationships." Journal of Bodywork and Movement Therapies 12 (2): 146-150.

Fritel, X., A. Fauconnier, G. Bader, M. Cosson, P. Debodinance, X. Deffieux, P. Denys, et al. 2010. "Diagnosis and Management of Adult Female Stress Urinary Incontinence: Guidelines for Clinical Practice From the French College of Gynaecologists and Obstetricians." *European Journal of Obstetrics and Gynecology and Reproductive Biology* 151 (1): 14-19.

Hagen, S., and D. Stark. 2011. "Conservative Prevention and Management of Pelvic Organ Prolapse in Women." The Cochrane Library.

Hernández-Gascón, B., A. Mena, E. Peña, G. Pascual, J.M. Bellón, and B. Calvo. 2013. "Understanding the Passive Mechanical Behavior of the Human Abdominal Wall." *Annals of Biomedical Engineering* 41 (2): 433-44.

Hodges, P.W. 1997. "Feedforward Contraction of Transversus Abdominis Is Not Influenced by the Direction of Arm Movement." *Experimental Brain Research* 114:362.

Hodges, P.W. 2011. "Pain and Motor Control: From the Laboratory to Rehabilitation." *Journal of Electromyography and Kinesiology* 21 (2): 220-8.

Hodges, P.W., J.E. Butler, D.K. McKenzie, and S.C. Gandevia. 1997. "Contraction of the Human Diaphragm During Rapid Postural Adjustments." *Journal of Physiology* 505 (2): 539.

Hodges, P.W., A. Kaigle Holm, S. Holm, L. Ekström, A. Cresswell, T. Hansson, and A. Thorstensson. 2003. "Intervertebral Stiffness of the Spine Is Increased by Evoked Contraction of Transversus Abdominis and the Diaphragm: In Vivo Porcine Studies." *Spine* 28 (23): 2594.

Hodges, P.W., R. Sapsford, and L.H.M. Pengel. 2007. "Postural and Respiratory Functions of the Pelvic Floor Muscles." *Neurourology and Urodynamics* 26 (3): 362.

Hungerford, B., W. Gilleard, and D. Lee. 2004. "Alteration of Pelvic Bone Motion Determined in Subjects With Posterior Pelvic Pain Using Skin Markers." *Clinical Biomechanics* 19 (5): 456-64.

Hungerford, B., W. Gilleard, M. Moran, and C. Emmerson. 2007. "Evaluation of the Ability of Physical Therapists to Palpate Intrapelvic Motion With the Stork Test on the Support Side." *Physical Therapy* 87 (7): 879-87.

Junginger, B., K. Baessler, R. Sapsford, and P.W. Hodges. 2010. "Effect of Abdominal and Pelvic Floor Tasks on Muscle Activity, Abdominal Pressure and Bladder Neck." *International Urogynecology Journal* 21 (1): 69-77.

Keeler, J., M. Albrecht, L. Eberhardt, L. Horn, C. Donnelly, and D. Lowe. 2012. "Diastasis Recti Abdominis: A Survey of Women's Health Specialists for Current Physical Therapy Clinical Practice for Postpartum Women." *Journal of Women's Health Physical Therapy* 36 (3): 131-42.

Lee, D. 2011. *The Pelvic Girdle: An Integration of Clinical Expertise and Research.* Edinburgh: Elsevier.

Lee, D., and P.W. Hodges. 2016. "Behavior of the Linea Alba During a Curl-Up Task in Diastasis Rectus Abdominis: An Observational Study." *Journal of Orthopaedic & Sports Physical Therapy* 46 (7): 580-89.

Lee, D.G., L.J. Lee, and L.M. McLaughlin. 2008. "Stability, Continence and breathing: The Role of Fascia Following Pregnancy and Delivery." *Journal of Bodywork and Movement Therapies* 12:333.

Liaw, L.J., M.J. Hsu, C.F. Liao, M.F. Liu, and A.T. Hsu. 2011. "The Relationships Between Inter-Recti Distance Measured by Ultrasound Imaging and Abdominal Muscle Function in Postpartum Women: A 6-Month Follow-Up Study." *Journal of Orthopaedic and Sports Physical Therapy* 41 (6): 435443.

Litos, K. 2014. "Progressive Therapeutic Exercise Program for Successful Treatment of a Postpartum Woman With a Severe Diastasis Recti Abdominis." *Journal of Women's Health Physical Therapy* 38 (2): 58-73.

Mason, D.J., D.K. Newman, and M.H. Palmer. 2003. "Changing UI Practice: This Report Challenges Nurses to Lead the Way in Managing Incontinence." *American Journal of Nursing* 103:2-3.

Mendes, D.D., F.X. Nahas, D.F. Veiga, F.V. Mendes, R.G. Figueiras, H.C. Gomes, P.B. Ely, et al. (2007). "Ultrasonography for Measuring Rectus Abdominis Muscles Diastasis." *Acta Cirúrgica Brasileira* 22 (3): 182-6.

Mørkved, S., and K. Bø. 2014. "Effect of Pelvic Floor Muscle Training During Pregnancy and After Childbirth on Prevention and Treatment of Urinary Incontinence: A Systematic Review." *British Journal of Sports Medicine* 48 (4): 299-310.

Mørkved, S., K. Bø, B. Schei, and K.A. Salvesen. 2003. "Pelvic Floor Muscle Training During Pregnancy to Prevent Urinary Incontinence: A Single-Blind Randomized Controlled Trial." *Obstetrics and Gynecology* 101 (2): 313-9.

Mottola, M. F., M.H. Davenport, C.R. Brun, S.D. Inglis, S. Charlesworth, and M.M. Sopper, 2006. "VO2peak Prediction and Exercise Prescription for Pregnant Women." *Medicine & Science in Sports & Exercise* 38(8): 1389-1395.

Noble, E. 1995. *Essential Exercises for the Childbearing Year: A Guide to Health and Comfort Before and After Your Baby Is Born.* Harwich, MA: New Life Images.

Nygaard, I.E., F.L. Thompson, S.L. Svengalis, and J.P. Albright. 1994. "Urinary Incontinence in Elite Nulliparous Athletes." *Obstetrics and Gynecology* 84 (2): 183-7.

Ostgaard, H.C., G.J. Andersson, and K. Karlsson. 1991. "Prevalence of Back Pain in Pregnancy." *Spine* 16:549-52.

Parker, M.A., L.A. Millar, and S.A. Dugan. 2009. "Diastasis Rectus Abdominis and Lumbo-Pelvic Pain and Dysfunction—Are They Related?" *Journal of Women's Health Physical Therapy* 33 (2): 15.

Pool-Goudzwaard, A.L., M.C. Slieker ten Hove, M.E. Vierhout, P.H. Mulder, J.J. Pool, C.J. Snijders, and R. Stoeckart. 2005. "Relations Between Pregnancy-Related Low Back Pain, Pelvic Floor Activity and Pelvic Floor Dysfunction." *International Urogynecology Journal* 16 (6): 468-74.

Rath, A.M., P. Attali, J.L. Dumas, D. Goldlust, J. Zhang, and J.P. Chevrel. 1996. "The Abdominal Linea Alba: An Anatomo-Radiologic and Biomechanical Study." *Surgical and Radiologic Anatomy* 18 (4): 281-8.

Rocha, J., P. Brandao, A. Melo, S. Torres, L. Mota, and F. Costa. 2017. "Assessment of Urinary Incontinence in Pregnancy and Postpartum: Observational Study." *Acta Médica Portuguesa* 30 (7-8): 568-72.

Röst, C.C., J. Jacqueline, A. Kaiser, A.P. Verhagen, and B.W. Koes. 2004. "Pelvic Pain During Pregnancy: A Descriptive Study of Signs and Symptoms of 870 Patients in Primary Care." *Spine* 29 (22): 2567-72.

Russell, J.G.B. 1982. "The Rationale of Primitive Delivery Positions." *British Journal of Obstetrics and Gynaecology* 89:712-5.

Salvatore, S., G. Siesto, and M. Serati. 2010. "Risk Factors for Recurrence of Genital Prolapse." *Current Opinion in Obstetrics and Gynecology* 22 (5): 420-4.

Sahrmann, S. 2001. *Diagnosis and Treatment of Movement Impaired Syndromes.* St. Louis: Mosby.

Sapsford, R.R., and P.W. Hodges. 2001. "Contraction of the Pelvic Floor Muscles During Abdominal Maneuver." *Archives of Physical Medicine & Rehabilitation* 82:1081.

Sapsford, R.R., P.W. Hodges, C.A. Richardson, D.H. Cooper, S.J. Markwell, and G.A. Jull. 2001. "Co-Activation of the Abdominal and Pelvic Floor Muscles During Voluntary Exercises." *Neurourology and Urodynamics* 20:31.

Signorello, L.B., B.L. Harlow, A.K. Chekos, and J.T. Repke. 2001. "Postpartum Sexual Functioning and Its Relationship to Perineal Trauma: A Retrospective Cohort Study of Primiparous Women." *American Journal of Obstetrics and Gynecology* 184 (5): 881-90.

Smith, M.D., A. Russell, and P.W. Hodges. 2006. "Disorders of Breathing and Continence Have a Stronger Association With Back Pain Than Obesity and Physical Activity." *The Australian Journal of Physiotherapy* 52 (2): 11-16.

Smith, M.D., A. Russell, and P.W. Hodges. 2008. "Is There a Relationship Between Parity, Pregnancy, Back Pain and Incontinence?" *International Urogynecology Journal and Pelvic Floor Dysfunction* 19 (2): 205-11.

Smith, M.D., A. Russell, and P.W. Hodges. 2014. "The Relationship Between Incontinence, Breathing Disorders, Gastrointestinal Symptoms and Back Pain in Women: A Longitudinal Cohort Study." *Clinical Journal of Pain* 30 (2): 162-7.

Society of Obstetricians and Gynecologists of Canada. 2003. "Exercise in Pregnancy and the Postpartum Period." Joint SOGC/CESP Clinical Practice Guideline, No. 129, June 2003. https://sogc.org/wp-content/uploads/2013/01/129E-JCPG-June2003.pdf.

Soma-Pillay, P., N.-P. Catherine, H. Tolppanen, A. Mebazaa, H. Tolppanen, and A. Mebazaa. 2016. "Physiological Changes in Pregnancy." *Cardiovascular Journal of Africa* 27 (2): 89-94.

Spitznagle, T.M., F.C. Leong, and L.R. Van Dillen. 2007. "Prevalence of Diastasis Recti Abdominis in a Urogynecological Patient Population." *International Urogynecology Journal* 18:321-8.

Viktrup, L., and G. Lose. 2000. "Lower Urinary Tract Symptoms 5 Years After the First Delivery." *International Urogynecology Journal and Pelvic Floor Dysfunction* 11 (6): 336-40.

Whiteside, J., A.M. Weber, L.A. Meyn, and M.D. Walters. 2004. "Risk Factors for Prolapse Recurrence After Vaginal Repair." *American Journal of Obstetrics and Gynecology* 191 (5): 1533-8.

Willard, F.H., A. Vleeming, M.D. Schuenke, L. Danneels, and R. Schleip. 2012. "The Thoracolumbar Fascia: Anatomy, Function and Clinical Considerations." *Journal of Anatomy* 221 (6): 507-36.

Wilson, P.D., P. Herbison, C. Glazener, M. McGee, and C. MacArthur. 2002. "Obstetric Practice and Urinary Incontinence 5-7 Years After Delivery." *ICS Proceedings Neurourology and Urodynamics* 21 (4): 284-300.

Wolfe, L.A., and M.F. Mottola. 2000. "Validations of Guidelines for Aerobic Exercise in Pregnancy." In *Decision Making and Outcomes in Sports Rehabilitation*, edited by D.A Kumbhare and J.V. Basmajian, 205-22. New York: Churchill Livingstone.

Wray, J. 2011."Bouncing Back? An Ethnographic Study Exploring the Context of Care and Recovery After Birth Through the Experiences and Voices of Mothers." PhD thesis, University of Salford, Salford, UK. https://my.rcn.org.uk/__data/assets/pdf_file/0008/459035/Wray_Julie_complete_thesis_2011.pdf.

Wu, W.H., O.G. Meijer, K. Uegaki, J.M. Mens, J.H. van Dieën, I.J. Wuisman, and H.C. Östgaard. 2004. "Pregnancy-Related Pelvic Girdle Pain (PPP): Terminology, Clinical Presentation, and Prevalence." *European Spine Journal* 13 (7): 575-89.

Zeelha, A., R. Thankar, and A.H. Sultan. 2009. "Postpartum Female Sexual Function: A Review." *European Journal of Obstetrics & Gynecology and Reproductive Biology* 145 (2): 133-7.

INDEX

Note: The italicized *f* and *t* following page numbers refer to figures and tables, respectively.

ABOUT THE AUTHORS

The authors are three highly qualified women's health professionals who are passionate about helping women improve their prenatal and postnatal fitness. After years of training individuals and running successful independent businesses, they started Bellies Inc., a global company dedicated to helping educate and empower women in their pregnancies, births, and recoveries. They bring to this book both their shared interest of helping women understand prenatal and postnatal fitness and their unique professional experience.

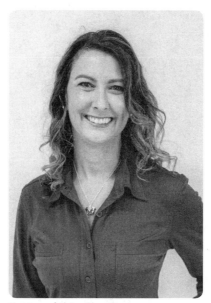

Courtesy of Elaine Chan-Dow.

Julia Di Paolo, Reg. PT, received her physiotherapy degree from the University of Ottawa in 1997. Her practice is focused on the preconception, prenatal, intrapartum (labor and delivery), and postpartum stages and on all types of pelvic floor dysfunction at any stage of a woman's life. Over the years, Di Paolo has established herself as the go-to physiotherapist in Toronto for pelvic health and recovery from diastasis rectus abdominis (DRA).

Di Paolo teaches courses on diastasis rectus abdominis for personal trainers, allied health professionals, and pelvic health physiotherapists. She has presented on DRA and the pelvic floor at the conferences of the Association of Ontario Midwives, the Ontario Physiotherapy Association, canfitpro, and the Certified Personal Trainer Network (CPTN, formerly Canadian Personal Trainers Network).

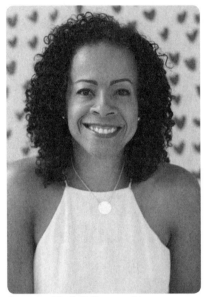

Courtesy of Emily D Photography.

Samantha Montpetit-Huynh received her fitness leadership certificate from Seneca College in 2002. She has been a personal trainer for over 15 years, focusing on pregnancy and postpartum fitness. She is also certified as a fitness for fertility specialist.

Samantha is known extensively in her field and has appeared on Breakfast Television, CTV News, Canada AM, CHCH, and Rogers Daytime. She was also the resident fitness expert on the Marilyn Denis Show, an award-winning lifestyle show seen across Canada, from 2013 to 2017. Samantha also helped to create the Today's Parent Healthy Pregnancy Guide.

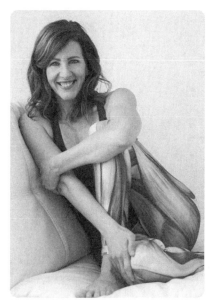

Courtesy of Photobin Photography.

Kim Vopni holds a bachelor's degree in psychology from the University of Western Ontario and a postgraduate diploma in health and fitness from Simon Fraser University. She has more than 15 years of skilled experience and is certified as a personal trainer, prenatal and postnatal fitness consultant, and fitness for fertility specialist. She is also a hypopressive method instructor. Kim is a passionate speaker, educator, and promoter of pelvic health and is known as the Vagina Coach.

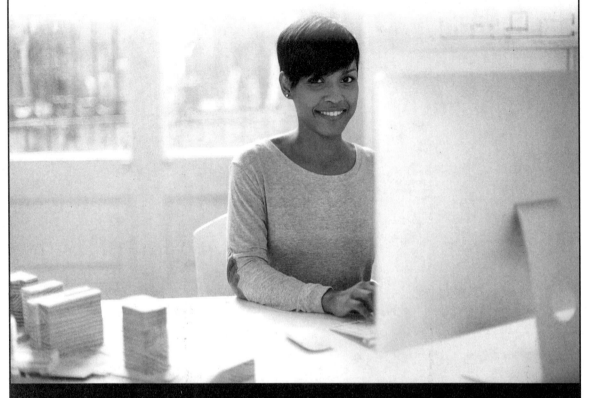
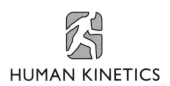